Parenting
a path through childhood

Dotty Turner Coplen

Parenting
a path
through
childhood

Floris Books

First published in 1982 by Floris Books
Reprinted 1988

© Dotty Turner Coplen, 1982

HQ
755.8
. C66
1982

British Library CIP Data available

ISBN 0-903540-61-4

Printed in Great Britain
at the University Printing House, Oxford

Contents

Contents

With thanks to the Reverend Walter Brecker and Sigfrid Knauer, MD, who have generously helped me on my search for truth and reality, and deep gratitude to the heritage of Rudolf Steiner.

1. Parenting today

Being a parent today is an awesome task. The demands are great and the expectations are high. The world is so full of information and ideas that it can overwhelm us rather than guide us. As parents we have to choose how to decide what authority or what theory we will follow. Who is right? As more and more professional literature on child care becomes available, a new dilemma presents itself. The theories are many and varied, sometimes contradictory, and parents are faced with the need to choose what theory to follow and when. For those of us attracted by a natural life style, combining scientific information with a natural philosophy is a difficult task.

It is my hope in this book to sort out some of the tangle of information; to select parenting methods compatible with the family life-style is essential. It also helps to know why you are doing things, what effect they will have, and how you decide.

We no longer live by strong traditions of what is right or wrong in child behaviour and child care. Although this provides some advantages, it also makes parenting a vast horizon of unknowns. Traditions which were originally developed out of an understanding of what was appropriate will have to be replaced by some other structure; we must replace them with new ways of understanding. Until we understand ourselves, our child, and our world in all its complexities, we cannot really make informed choices. Somewhere we have to find a starting-point for establishing some basic realities in in this world of illusion, fantasy, and deception. We need to find theories that we can observe and evaluate to help us understand our relationships to each other, our children and the world. It is as important to know *what* we are doing and *why*, as it is to know *how* to do it.

The fuller the bookshelves become with books on child care, child development, behaviour management, and parent-child relationships, the more difficult it becomes to sort out the good theories from the bad. Living in the world has become more and more complex as industry has created more time and labour-saving devices. Many people are at a loss to find their place in the world and make some sense out of life. When children ask 'why?' it gets harder and harder to find a real answer.

The family traditions that formerly supported the social structure are disappearing. The concept of hierarchy authority (that the wise, the powerful, the good will make the appropriate decisions for themselves and others) is no longer believed. People think for themselves, reject being used, or told what to do, and although people know what they don't want, it is another thing to know what they do want. What is the ideal way of life? Without an ideal, how can we evaluate what is happening? Without some criteria for judgment, how do we know if new solutions are right or wrong, kind or unkind, reasonable or unreasonable?

As the void created by loss of tradition grows larger, science produces more and more options such as life-saving techniques, life-sustaining possibilities, euthanasia, nuclear weapons, birth control, artificial fabrics, plastic materials, artificial flavours, and so on. With the ability to create man-made substances and machine-made goods, we have created polluting by-products, energy shortages and less need for manpower, fewer jobs, and contempt for those who do not work (unless they are rich). Do we need more people or fewer people, or should man be making that decision for his fellow man? We have created new moral, ethical problems as we have progressed scientifically. Is science to be the ruler or servant of man? If we do not understand what is happening around us and where we are going, we live life as victims in the world.

A valuable source of wisdom for approaching these problems comes from the works of Rudolf Steiner. An Austrian philosopher-scientist, he devoted his life to bringing true knowledge into science, art, religion and to bringing them into their right relationship with each other. He asked that his thoughts not be taken as true because he said them, but that they be taken as possibilities, to be proved or disproved by one's own experience. His contribution to a new understanding of the world and the creatures living in it is immense. His writings include philosophy, psychology, art, science, religion and indications for practical endeavours such as education, medicine, gardening, economics, political life, social life, and so on.

One of his contributions is a new way of

understanding man. He develops the concept of man as a being with capacities for thinking, feeling and willing, and an ego which allows him to choose how he will use these capacities. To understand ourselves and our fellow man in this way allows us to observe the concepts that we are working with rather than accept abstract dogma. By carefully observing ourselves and others we come to know man in this way.

First we have thinking. We can use the concept of thinking in a general way to include learning information, discovering ideas, and knowing about the world by using our thought processes. The capacity for thinking we are given, the information about the world we gain as we learn.

Next we identify feeling, how we feel about things. Through feeling we relate to things we like and do not like; how we react to the world. Feelings are a very personal matter and we can learn to control and change them.

Then we understand will in relation to activity, doing things, both starting and stopping. Finally we have the ego, the 'I' in us. It is the individual part of each person: *I* think, *I* like, *I* walk. Our personality is determined by the interrelationship of our thinking, our feeling, and our willing. It is with our ego that we can accept or reject what we are doing, thinking or feeling and alter that. With our ego we act rather than react. If this sounds complex, let me assure you that it is not. It may be a new way of thinking; but all these aspects are part of you and can be experienced by you. You can learn about and understand this phenomenon in a really practical way on a daily basis because it is you. Just as the child learns to know the world from those around him, we can learn to understand the world by observing ourselves, each other and our children, and by listening.

The current generation of parents, like those before them, are faced with many opportunities and many pitfalls. Although the kinds of problems and choices remain similar throughout history, the degrees of difference seem to be of greater magnitudes. We have an ever-increasing number of choices. Because we can do something does not mean that doing it is inevitable or right. Even though we have the capability of blowing up the whole earth and destroying it, that does not mean that we have to choose to do that. It matters more and more what choices and decisions we make and how well we do things. It is my hope that the ideas presented here will help you with your choices.

2. A child is born

When a child is born, a world of wonder is brought into our lives. We sense the thrill of a new beginning, rather like an early morning sunrise. The wonder and wisdom of nature are made visible. Fortunate are the mother and father who have prepared together for the birth of their child as a conscious, shared experience. They are living through one of the wonders of the world. Awe and reverence are inevitable for those who have looked at the creation of their baby with an attempt at understanding.

From conception, through the first moments of feeling your baby move, to the eventual vigorous kicking, the stages of labour, the delivery, and the first sight of your baby, you come to know that the world beyond human control is working. The world we cannot count or measure, and yet is obviously there.

Fortunate is the baby whose parents allow this process to unfold in a natural way, neither feeling the need to control the time of birth for their convenience, nor allowing the time to be controlled for the doctor's convenience. If we really recognize the magnitude of this miracle of nature, we can prepare for it in a beautiful way, aware of the effects on the baby. By directing our thoughts and efforts toward allowing the baby to be born at the time and in the way that is best for him, we are not tempted to be clever or controlling. Rather we attempt to co-operate with and understand what is happening. We realize that baby, too, will experience this event.

We avoid being bewildered by over-simplified yet complicated scientific theories that think only in terms of brain and nervous system function and we realize that the brain is only part of the baby's body and life. There is also the heart, the liver, the lungs, the spleen, the glands, the sun, the stars, the planets, the moon, the air, the mother, the father and much, much more. By being aware of the relationships and interactions of all aspects of the world and the cosmos, we shall be saved from the one-sidedness that prevents true understanding. We do not let the process and details and method obscure the important fact that a child is being born. Through the laws of nature and the wisdom of the world a new baby has been conceived, grown and developed and a new life will start, unlike any other. To try to comprehend what that experience will be for her we can call on our memory and try with our imagination to develop an understanding of what is happening.

Try to remember sitting in a room with the lights out, a fire burning in the fireplace, and perhaps a beeswax candle or two as the only other light in the room. We experience warmth and gentleness. We feel calm, relaxed and harmonious. For the moment we forget the cares and demands of the world and live in this pleasant moment of softness and gentleness. We relish the moment of escape. Then someone new comes into the room, talking loudly and turning on all the electric lights. What a shock! We experience it as a shock. The electric lights and the noise seem hard and cold and attacking. If you can't remember such an experience, try it and see. Then you will have an inkling of what it must be like for a new-born baby. She comes from a warm, protected, nourishing environment into a world where she must find air to breathe, food to digest, and maintain her own warmth. Her body must learn to function independently. She is faced with a dramatic change from the warm, safe world that she experienced before birth to this new unprotected environment. Knowing this, we try to minimize the trauma. We make the change as gentle as possible. We seek professional care from those who share this knowledge of the importance of the surroundings throughout pregnancy and at the time of birth.

Before birth the child is protected from the outer environment; she is living in the environment of the mother. It is the mother who provides the feeling of soft candle-light or of hard electric lights for the baby. Mother creates the environment. Our body reflects our emotions. We know that when we are embarrassed, we blush, when we are frightened we pale. Those are physical manifestations of feelings. The way we feel affects our physical body. When we are excited our heart beats faster, when we are angry we have knots in our stomach and don't feel like eating. Differing emotions bring about different body conditions. The baby's breathing and nutrition and circulation are united with the mother's and there is no escape. The bodily changes in the mother will inevitably be reflected in the baby.

16

Fathers too have an important role before the birth of their baby. Fathers recognize the importance of helping mother to provide the optimum nurturing environment for their baby. Both parents recognize the importance of the father's role throughout the pregnancy as well as at the time of birth. It is father who makes it possible for mother to feel protected and cared for so that together they can provide nurturing harmony for their child. It does matter a lot what goes on emotionally as well as physically during the time of pregnancy. This is a shared task for mother and father. They both matter, and matter a lot. The child is not an inanimate object or an island. She absorbs and is affected by everything that surrounds her.

After she is born, she trusts that her parents will give her milk, the warmth, the protection from noise and confusion that she needs. She trusts that they will provide a serene and caring environment. She needs parents who will care enough.

This tiny one brings about oh's and ah's as we experience her delicateness and the need for gentleness that come to us as we care for her. If it is our first experience with a baby, we may stand back a bit, amazed, not sure how to approach this tiny bundle.

While baby sleeps there is an air of mystery surrounding her and instinctively we speak in hushed tones. Parents are calm and baby is warm and full; sleep is her priority. A feeling of awe and warmth and love seem to accompany a baby; somehow she nurtures and inspires those around who care for her. Despite the startling experience of being born, baby trusts that those around will care for her. And parents do perform remarkable deeds of sacrifice as they care for their little one.

When baby becomes hungry, she wakes; cries to alert those whom she trusts will bring the necessary milk. It will be mother's milk from mother's breast if she has the best of all worlds. When parents are attuned and reading the subtle cues from their baby, all goes well, and having a baby is a delightful experience for all concerned.

But babies are complex biological organisms and reading the cues is not a simple task. Harmony and contentment are not the only realities in babies' lives. When all is not well, baby starts to fuss, she is uncomfortable, and with this, our experience also changes. The feelings of light and warmth are replaced by doubt, concern, maybe apprehension. Those not responsible for her care say, with a barely detectable tone of relief, 'She wants her mother or dad.' You as the parent are faced with the task of discovering the cause of the change and also the cure. It is obvious that baby is trying to tell you something, but what? Now it is up to you. You must meet baby's gift to you of joy and warmth with your gift of care. Communication is difficult.

Your baby asks you to care for her and somehow you must develop the necessary capacities to discover the baby's needs and how to meet them. Is she hungry, wet, cold, hot, in pain? What is it? What does she want? We consider all possibilities. We change her, we dress her appropriately, not too warm or too cold, we make sure the room is not too noisy or too bright. We wrap her in a blanket so that she can feel protected and then feed her warm milk, all the while trying to remain calm. And if all goes well we are back to harmony and contentment.

It is during these very moments, early in the baby's life, that she learns about the world. This is the meeting of the baby's world with the outer world, her new environment. Out of the meeting of these two worlds arises the beginning of life's experiences.

The child comes into our world with warmth, love and trust, qualities that we also cherish in an adult. The nature of the baby comes with her and lives in her. We don't make it or put it there. She is not an empty vessel to be filled, but a being to be recognized and experienced. These qualities live, and how they develop is affected by us. The way we care for her does affect her development.

How can we keep this warmth, love and trust alive for this little one? When we meet an adult who is warm, friendly, and understanding, we enjoy being with him and feel that he is somehow special. Yet these qualities are gifts from birth. How can we preserve them? Can we find what it is that allows this humanness, these qualities of warmth and love to remain through childhood to adulthood. We know what we experience from the child. Can we imagine what the child experiences? What can we really know about — not out of theory, but out of our own observation? Can we know from her what is necessary, what is important?

Perhaps we can try to understand what it must be like to be a baby. She must have feelings or she wouldn't be alternately smiling, fussing and crying. What she feels she seems to experience in her whole body. We take off her clothes in a cool room, she cries as she gets chilled. She wakes from her nap and cries because she is hungry. A sudden loud noise and she cries. When she cries her arms and legs move, she gets red in the face and she cries with her whole body.

We put her clothes on and she gets warm, we feed her and she is full, the crying stops, the body quietens down and relaxes and if we speak softly to her she smiles at us. What does this tell us? What can we learn from this?

The baby feels, and expresses her feelings. She feels the comforts and discomforts of her body. She does not think, 'I am cold and I'm going to make them do something about it'. But she feels her distress and calls to us by crying, trusting that we will find the cause and help her. She is unable to help herself. She needs parents to care for her. By crying she lets us know that she feels discomfort. When she smiles, it is with her whole body: she wiggles all over. When she cries, it is also a total show: arms, legs, mouth and eyes. For the baby there are no words and no thoughts to sort out and communicate. She doesn't 'know' where she hurts or what is causing it. But feel it she does. She is totally dependent on someone else to sort out what is causing her discomfort; to make her warm and dry and full and comfortable again, to protect her and care for her, to return the love and delight that she so freely gives. Her needs and demands of us are as great as her gifts to us.

We can see how eagerly the child anticipates being

held and how she enjoys the touch and warmth of a caring person. If the child has the good fortune of being cared for according to her own needs, then often her fussing will stop when she is picked up. This does not mean that she is spoiled, but rather that she trusts those who care for her. She has learned that the person who comes to her will provide what she needs. One of the parents' tasks is to develop a sense for knowing what is making the baby unhappy. Is she cold, is she wet, is she hungry, or is she lonely? If she is cold and you feed her, she may enjoy eating, but she is still cold. She will continue to fuss. For the parent as well as the child it is an experience of getting to know another person as she really is. Not as we want her to be, but as she really is.

In these early months we become aware that baby is wise beyond words. She knows when there is harmony and when there is disharmony for her. She experiences it and relates this experience to us. We can learn what she needs if we can really learn to 'listen' to her, not just hear her crying and cooing, but listen beyond words and sounds to what is being communicated.

Babies differ from an early age in how they communicate. Some are persistent, others give up easily, some are loud, others soft-spoken, some are robust, some more delicate, some are more alert and others dreamy. Differences that become more obvious as the child grows older are there from the beginning for those who develop the capacity to observe the subtle cues. If we learn to know the baby as she really is then we enable her to come into the world with a feeling of acceptance. For this to happen, a great deal of appropriate parenting has to occur. Different children have different needs and the same approach will not work with all children. Beware of those who stand in judgment and tell you that you are not a good parent and your child is bad. Good and bad are words that have very little value in parenting. They are based on arbitrary expectations that have nothing to do with understanding your child, her needs in the world and appropriate ways to meet them. They do not lead us closer to our goal of providing appropriate care for a child.

Children, unlike animals, are born totally incapable of caring for themselves. They are unable to move to find their source of food, they do not have a furry covering to keep them warm. They are totally exposed to their environment and dependent on their parents to provide and care for them. This asks of the parents the ability first to recognize and understand the child's needs and then be willing to provide for them, not only when the parent feels like it, but all the time — certainly, one of life's most demanding tasks.

Babies, like flowers, have to have the elements necessary for their growth brought to them. Babies are obviously more than flowers and yet there are common needs. They are both dependent on food, drink, warmth and light being brought to them to allow them to grow and develop. Some children are bright and cheery like daisies and daffodils, some are beautiful like roses, some are sturdy like oaks, some are whimsical like wildflowers. The varieties in all of nature are immense; in flowers, trees, animals and most of all in people. Just as we would not criticize a daisy for not being a rose, or judge one to be better than another, our baby needs us to accept and acknowledge who she is and help her to unfold those qualities that are uniquely hers.

But babies are more than flowers and they need to move. This wisdom is also in babies. Early in their life, on their own, they make what appear to be random movements. As the child develops, the random movements slowly become purposeful and controlled movements. Baby's hand clasps a finger, hand touches hand, baby lifts her head, and slowly establishes the ability to use her body. As we watch the child grow we see the forces of nature unfold within the child. She eats and digests, she breathes, she is warm-blooded, she moves about. She grows and develops. Things we also see happening in the animals and in the plants.

But in man there are other qualities that we do not see anywhere else in nature. Qualities that are uniquely human also unfold. Baby has to develop these qualities too. There is the beginning of speech—individually formed sounds that will be combined into words to convey meanings, to communicate thoughts and ideas.

How amazingly different is the spoken human word from animal sounds: what variety and what possibilities.

Baby also relentlessly pursues being upright in the world: first lifting the head, then lifting the trunk so that she learns to sit and then to stand upright, finally she learns to walk. Nowhere else in nature do we see this develop in the same way. All these abilities are being formed, developed and worked on in the first year of the baby's life. A large task for this little one. What she eats, who she is with, and where she is will all have some effect on this development.

The child stands up in the world and walks. Again there are differences. Children use their bodies differently. Some children glide swiftly like deer, some move more ceremoniously like cows, some are born natural climbers like sure-footed goats, some dart about like mice, some are as agile as cats. Still one is not better than the other. They are different and variety is the spice of life and the gift of nature.

The child stands up in the world and walks. She goes through the world upright and her hands and arms are free for her to use. Because of that she is able to live a life that is uniquely human. She can learn to write, draw, build furniture, make pottery, jewellery, farm equipment, the endless list that differentiates man's social and cultural world from the natural environment. Whether or not it is done wisely and well is up to man; but the ability to do so is a uniquely human gift.

3. Creating his world

As your baby grows and your role as parent becomes more defined, you face some inevitable decisions. As you proceed with the task of parenting, your basic philosophies of life will be lived. You may not even consciously know what your philosophy is, but you will be working out of it, rather like the child who said, 'Let me talk about it so I can hear what I think.'

Your philosophy may come from what the world has taught you about life and that may not be what you want to live out of. Perhaps you want your child's life to be different from yours in some ways. If you haven't stopped to consider before what your priorities are and what matters, now is a good time to take a look. What kind of parent do you want to be? Where will you look for direction and alternatives? Whose advice do you seek? Of all the 'experts' in the world, which do you choose to follow? Where do you find out how to be a parent and make the choices that you want to make? The world seems to be full of 'how to' books on almost every subject we can think of. If you want to make a dress, a table, a garden, raise chickens, or whatever, you are certain to find adequate instructions. We can also read 'how to' win friends, be a better salesman, succeed in college and anything else we want to learn. If the first book we read and follow does not give us a satisfactory product or

25

experience, we can always find a better set of directions and try again. However, with children, if part way through the process of parenting we find our instructions were not appropriate, we cannot go back to the beginning of the child's life and start again. We have to go on from where we are. Childhood cannot be started again. We can change to different ways, but what has gone before is real and inevitably the effects will be there. That is not to discourage us, but to let us know that what we do matters.

Since the effects on plants are more visible because they develop in a shorter space of time, we will use an example from the plant world. We realize our child is much more than a plant but we will use the analogy as a way of understanding causality.

We plant a daisy in a pot, care for it until it sprouts. After it has grown an inch or so, we tip the pot at forty-five degrees. Amazingly the plant will right itself as it grows so that it will grow straight out toward the sun, away from the earth's force of gravity. It will grow and flower despite the tipped pot. However, the stem will have a forty-five degree bend one inch up from the ground. Now we have not changed the inherent quality or character of the daisy; its nature is still there and it has fulfilled its life cycle, but it has a bend in the stem that it had to develop to compensate for our action. Whether or not this weakens the plant depends on how vital the seed was, how fertile the soil was, how much sun and moisture it had.

And so it is with the child. We are not the all-controlling force and power in the child's life. The world wisdom and nature forces are stronger, but we can be an enabler or a hindrance. What we do will affect the unfolding or inhibiting of the nature and talents of the child. Avoiding errors through some forethought is a much more rewarding process than lamenting over our errors and the consequences of them.

There are books on baby care you can refer to. Some will tell you to feed the baby when he is hungry, some will tell you to establish a schedule and stick to it, some will suggest you let the baby cry for five minutes and if after five minutes he is still crying, feed him. Neighbours, grandparents, aunts, uncles, doctors, nurses, will all be glad to give you their advice and suggestions. Early in the parenting role you are forced to make a decision as to what method you will follow, or what advice you will take. If you decide not to decide, that is also a decision. If you have a basis for making these extremely important decisions, then parenting can become a rewarding life's task.

Perhaps, 'how to' be a parent should not be the first question that a parent asks. As you start into the amazing adventure of being a parent, before finding out 'how to' it seems necessary first to explore *what* is a parent and *why* does a child need one. So let's try.

Where do we start to explore *what* is a parent? We ask ourselves the question and find we already know some answers. The parent cares for the child, feeds the child and protects the child. Depending on where we live and what our life style is we may teach manners and respect, we may discipline or punish. But

27

knowing that these are some of the responsibilities of parenting really isn't a lot of help in the day to day process of parenting. Perhaps we need a clearer view of *who* a child is. We can also answer that. As a baby at least, a child is a helpless little one, at times hungry or fussy, a lot of work, a delight to be around when his needs are satisfied and he is happy; a frustrating experience when he cries and we don't know why. A baby is in a world that he can't cope with on his own. He needs someone to care for his bodily needs and to allow him to feel cared for, safe and secure.

Once we realize the total dependence of a baby, it is fairly easy to find out *why* he needs a parent. It is obvious that babies are helpless in some very basic ways. They can't go for food when they are hungry, they can't cover themselves when they are cold and they can't dry themselves when they are wet. Those are some of the reasons *why* babies need parents.

But isn't it remarkable that a baby tells us when he needs to eat, when he is full, and we never taught him that. Some things children are born knowing and we can learn from them. We don't need to teach them to cry or to smile, to move their arms and legs, to see, to listen, to feel, to be happy or to be sad. All that knowing is already there for this little one. To feel and to move are God-given attributes that do not depend on learning.

Some experts will tell you that blind babies never smile. That is what other experts taught them in school. This is based on the assumption that a baby is an empty pitcher that must be filled, or an evolved animal that must be humanized, and therefore has to learn how to smile through imitation. If baby sees his mother smile, they say, he learns to smile. Since a blind baby never sees another smile, he can't learn how to smile. However, parents who have given warmth and loving care to their baby can tell you that their blind baby does smile.

That leads us back to the quandary of trying to decide what expert to follow and whose advice to take. It also gives us one clue. If we become careful observers of the world, we have that way to learn. True knowledge comes when what someone has told us corresponds with what we observe. Only then do we know out of our own experience what is true.

The world is remarkably full of information. The problem is that all the information is not totally true. It may be true part of the time in some situations, but when it is presented as a total truth it becomes untrue. Some blind babies don't smile, but the cause is not that they can't learn to smile because they can't see a smile. The effect is there, but the wrong cause is given. By telling parents that their child will never smile a barrier is placed between the parent and the child. The parent has misinformation that he will inevitably act out of.

When possible, the best thing to do with information is to take it only as a possibility and see if it checks out in your experience. This not only gives you the opportunity to sort out fact from fiction, but it also makes life an exciting game of discovery. The keener your ability is to observe the world, the richer it becomes and the more you can learn. It is through observing your child that you can learn the most about him. Of course observation must be done without preconceived ideas or prejudices. Not to prove that you know, but rather to discover what is true. What can you discover about your baby?

He tells us he knows how to feel. Stick a pin in him and he cries; he feels it. When he is hungry, he cries; he feels it. When he is fed and warm and cared for he smiles; he feels love. He receives love and he gives love. We feel it too. Through these feelings he can communicate with us and we can communicate with him. This is the beginning of his getting to know the world and expressing himself in the world. This early communication is an important experience. It is the early basis on which speech will later be built. To communicate to others and have them listen is the beginning of human interaction in the world.

Although he is totally aware of his own bodily needs, his comfort and his discomfort, he is equally helpless in providing the solutions to these discomforts. He feels that he is here in the world and the world impinges on him. He may be bothered by cold air, bright lights, loud noises, anxious parents, annoying pokes from exploring children or being put in a separate part of the house by himself. He is pleased by being close to another person, if they are enjoying his closeness; by warm milk in his hungry tummy, by feeling warm and safe. Not only is he pleased by feelings of bodily comfort, he expects them. Out of his own amazing wisdom he knows that it is important to take good care of his bodily needs and that a feeling of well-being is the state to be desired and achieved. He also experiences himself as someone who needs to be acknowledged, communicated with, and included in his parents' consciousness.

The baby can let you know when he is satisfied and that is a pleasant experience for all. He can let us know when all is not well. How the parents respond to these calls and messages from the child is the beginning of his learning about the physical world. The child experiences his own inner feelings of comfort and discomfort and experiences the emotional climate that his demands creates. Does the parent coldly and disinterestedly disregard the child because the mechanical clock on the wall says the baby does not need to eat? Who said the clock knows? Before he was born he was continually nourished. Now he needs time to learn to adapt to the idea of intermittent eating.

For him what he feels is true. Through our interaction with him, we teach him what to do with his feelings and his separateness. How he responds throughout his life to his feelings depends on how we respond to him. How do we react when he lets us know how he feels? Through what he is born knowing, and how we react to this knowing, he forms his personality.

If he is cared for in a reasonable way, if his needs are met most of the time, if he has loving people around, he will trust the world that he has joined. As he grows up, this trust in the world will develop into a trust in himself and he will have the necessary inner strength to meet the world with courage. He will have the possibility of knowing that whatever challenges his life may bring, somehow he will be able to meet them.

If he sometimes has to wait a bit, that will help him learn that others have needs too and he isn't the only one in the world to be considered. Don't expect him to like it though. His primary concern is surviving in this world and he doesn't have the ability to reason. It is through our reason, not our desires, that we learn to consider others. It is important he learns that not all his desires will be met or he will become a tyrant and that is not our goal as a parent. As he grows older it will be important that he learns impulse control and the basis of that learning can occur in infancy.

We don't have to teach him how to feel or that he is a unique individuality, we only have to accept and acknowledge that it is so.

For a child to develop a feeling of trust it is necessary for his world to be predictable and rhythmic. If there is a rhythm in the day, he will eventually learn to anticipate what will come next and feel secure and reassured when this happens. He will have the experience of recognizing the world and then he will feel a little safer in this large complicated place. We create a predictable world, a path, for him so that the bewildering and sometimes threatening and hostile world does not come too close when he is young. We use our strength and power to protect and care for him and guide him on this path through life.

Consistency and rhythm are important ingredients in the life of a child. In matters as simple as his bath we can provide this for him. First we wash his face, then his right arm, then his left arm, then his trunk, or whatever sequence we decide upon. If we always do this in the same order, eventually he will anticipate what is to be washed next and he will offer the arm or leg. Then he will experience that he and whoever baths him, both know the same thing. That is also a good experience. When we share our observations with others we don't feel so separate. As he becomes older he can use this same sequence to bath himself. Although we provide this rhythmic consistency for him to learn by, we don't tell him that it is *the* way to bath or demand that he use the sequence. We are merely providing a pattern for him to learn through. We are making the world consistent for the purpose of learning about it. By doing things in the same way we allow the world to become familiar.

It is possible to observe the child's appreciation of the familiar. Repetition delights him. He enjoys having the same songs sung to him, hearing the same sounds. Repetition is a basis for learning; and learning about the world around us gives an inner stability and feeling of comfort. It is much easier to relax in a familiar situation than it is when we don't know what to expect next. If each day is different, if he can't learn to count on the order in the day, then the child feels anxious and vulnerable.

Perhaps we can have a better understanding of this if we think of an adult situation that might compare. Let us imagine that you have moved to a foreign country where you cannot understand the language that is spoken. Further you have no place to buy and prepare your own food. You go to a restaurant for breakfast, are warmly greeted, and served a delightful breakfast. The next day no matter what you do or say this same restaurant will only give you coffee. The third day they will give you a delicious breakfast. The fourth day they shout at you and refuse to serve you any food. What will you expect on the fifth day? Will you go back for breakfast? You know it is the only place where you will be able to eat, but is it worth it? Well, you are hungry. How you respond will depend on your other life experiences and your own temperament. At the very least you will feel apprehensive — some people will feel totally bewildered and overwhelmed, some will feel angry.

We are learning from our experiences all the time and this is also true for children. Are the experiences that we are giving the child teaching him what we want him to learn about us and the world? As adults we function best when we have two elements in our life: rhythm most of the time; and on occasion, special events. For the young child the need is primarily for rhythm. Rhythm relates to sequence and dependability, not to a rigid routine. It doesn't mean that at exactly 7.00 you have a bottle and are allowed only ten minutes to drink it; or at precisely 9.00 you have a bath that takes exactly ten minutes. It doesn't mean being controlled by a clock or some dogma.

It does mean being consistent and dependable; one event follows another at approximately the same time in an ordered way. Rhythm lives in nature; our breathing is rhythmic, our heart beat is rhythmic. It is not always the same, but it is always rhythmic. The rhythm is slower when we sleep and faster when we exercise. The sun rises and sets in rhythm — the time changes a bit each day but it is an event that we can anticipate and count on. Lest you worry that this will make for a rigid, inflexible child, let us look a bit further into our imaginary experience.

If instead of the unpredictable restaurant situation that we found daily, we found that every morning we could have breakfast there, eventually we would be confident about getting breakfast and it wouldn't be a primary concern. We could then start learning about other things in this new area and we might even find another place to have breakfast. On our own we would find another way to do it. We would be feeling confident and perhaps adventuresome as we explored the other possibilities. If we looked for a new place out of bewilderment and confusion we would be apprehensive and perhaps resentful while we searched. It is through knowing and understanding the world that we can feel safe in it. By feeling safe in our world we can venture forth to learn to understand more of the world.

As parents we can create a recognizable path through childhood and then through life for the child. If the path is clearly defined, consistent, protected without being rigidly controlled, then in later years the child will be able to wander with confidence through life to experience other paths.

Baby loves rhythm in movement as well as in the daily schedule. We can observe the child's pleasure in rhythm, by his response to being rocked. He enjoys being rocked in his cradle, if he is so lucky as to have one, or in a rocking chair. If neither of these is available, it is still possible when holding him to move him in a gently swaying rocking movement. Rhythm is a dependable part of nature and babies are still closely linked with nature. Most babies develop an eating and sleeping rhythm after a few weeks in this world. Rhythm in eating is important for the baby, as is rhythm in sleeping. As much as possible the attempt should be made to discover and then maintain these rhythms. If the baby's natural rhythm doesn't fit into the family's rhythm then you can work at modifying it by degrees to make them compatible.

Warmth is another important experience for baby, both physical warmth and inner warmth, the experience of closeness and warmth of his parents. An infant is not able to maintain his own warmth and here too baby is dependent on those who care for him to provide adequate clothing and blankets for him to keep warm. A baby is not born being able to resist the environmental elements. We need to protect him. Happily, the philosophy of 'toughening' the baby has mostly disappeared. It became apparent that warmth and flexibility were qualities that serve us better for life and health. Being cold and tough does not lead to human understanding. Man is a warm-blooded creature and maintaining the proper warmth is important to good health. This can be done by dressing baby in natural fabrics; cottons and wools. Synthetic fabrics are not the same. Unfortunately, the longer we wear synthetic fabrics, the less discrimination we have. When synthetics were first made, people were aware that air could not pass through the fabric as it does in a natural fabric. Then people noticed the difference. They objected to the lack of absorbent qualities in synthetic fabrics. Our skin is also an organ of respiration and this is affected by synthetics. People were aware that the synthetic 'cottons' were uncomfortably warm in the summer and the synthetic 'wools' did not keep them warm in the winter. Natural materials relate to people; there is an exchange between the clothes and the people wearing them. Now people have worn synthetic fabrics for so long it has become much more difficult to discriminate. Part of the wonder of the human organism is that it will adapt to its environment and learn to cope with it. However, it is always at some cost. The effect of synthetic materials is difficult to experience and observe — but it is not impossible. Put a synthetic blanket over your face and breathe: notice that you feel suffocated? Now try a wool or cotton blanket. Notice the difference. When baby is in synthetic sleepers you may find that his skin is cold to the touch, but he is perspiring. Try him in cotton or wool sleepers and check the difference.

Try wearing only natural fabrics yourself for six months and then wear synthetic fabrics and see the difference for yourself. Static electricity is a problem with synthetic fabrics that you will not have with natural fabrics. The synthetic is a barrier; it does not absorb, transfer and conduct. It does not support the natural life processes. Synthetics do not appear in nature, they are man-made. This may lead you on a slight detour, because finding clothes of natural materials is not easy. The petrochemical industry has a strong hold on the world market and it is apparent in fabrics and fabric control. You may end up taking a sewing course, if you haven't already acquired this rewarding skill.

As baby grows stronger it is important that his clothing allows for freedom of movement. Moving about is another natural ability that baby has. First the seemingly random movement of the arms and legs, then the lifting of his head while on his tummy, then the supporting of his own head while being held. Eventually sitting, crawling, standing and walking. We don't have to teach baby to do this, but we do have to provide an opportunity for this natural development to unfold. It is interesting to observe how this physical development progresses in an orderly manner from the head to the toes. First he moves the head, then the neck, then the trunk and finally the legs. The baby will develop according to his own timetable if we provide the opportunity for it. As a newborn we must support his head when we hold him. As he grows stronger we give him the opportunity to hold his own head and to learn the beginning of balance. If he spends all his time lying in a crib, he will not be able to develop strength in his trunk. We need to give him the opportunity to sit up first with our support, and eventually on his own.

His random arm and leg movements will become co-ordinated into a crawling motion if he is allowed to be on the floor and given a chance to develop this ability. By occasionally having something for his feet to push against, such as his parent's hand, he develops this sense of where his feet are and what is going on with these movements. There is increasing evidence that the laterality that is learned through crawling, that is the co-ordination of the right hand, left foot, and left hand, right foot enhances the development of the nervous system that is later needed for reading.

By the end of the first year, baby will have mastered finding his place in space and will be able to stand. That is no easy task as it means he has to maintain a balance of front-back, up-down, and right-left. A bit too far in any direction and over he goes. There is no better example of indomitable courage in the world than the constant repeated efforts of a child learning to walk. After a fall he is up to try again until he succeeds. Giving up never occurs to him.

It is interesting to note that animals do not have to go through this lengthy process of developing the ability to walk. It is an innate ability that they have shortly after birth. It is also true that it is uniquely human to have the opportunity to walk totally upright, and to have two hands which are remarkably different from their two feet. Baby has to learn to walk in this special upright balance; the ability is not there at birth.

Baby's skull is not completely developed at birth either. In the first year of his life we need to be aware that the brain is not protected in the same way as it is in later life. Nature has carefully enclosed the brain in a strong bony skull, but in the young child this development is not finished. There are portions of the brain that are not covered by the skull, they are traditionally called 'soft spots'. Therefore, the head must be protected until the time the natural shield is completed. We need to protect the baby's head from bumps and also from the heat of the sun and cool wind. When baby goes outside in his early years he needs a cap or bonnet. Once the skull is closed and the brain has a complete covering it is less critical, although still important. The strong heat of the sun and cold wind penetrate the child and we have to be careful to protect him from extreme exposures. The brain must be a delicate fragile organ or nature would not have covered it with such sturdy protection and until this is there, we will have to take extra precautions.

All that goes on around the baby is taken in by him. Calm activity provides him with sense impressions that arouse his interest, but do not overwhelm him. When things are done with care and attentiveness he experiences an important human quality. It is living with caring people in a caring environment that brings to light our humanness. When we do the extra things that matter, we go beyond the world of drives, instincts, impulses, to the world of culture and morality.

Baby enjoys being around people and seeing movement. He enjoys being held by his parents and experiencing their warmth. Carrying baby is a natural occurrence since he has no mobility of his own: he has to be carried. However, if he is carried in a plastic baby carrier he is not having the experience of being held by his parents. The plastic is a barrier between the baby and his parents. This may not be so noticeable to the parents, but it is very noticeable to baby. Feeling hard, cold plastic is very different from experiencing the physical touching of his parents and their warmth.

Baby seats have their uses and it is a convenient piece of equipment to have, but be aware of what the baby experiences when he is in one. Do let him have the experience of being held and carried by you.

The environment is an important factor in the early experience of the child. This does not reduce the importance of heredity. What the child can do with his inherited qualities is influenced by his environment. His heredity and the effects of his environment are both modified by his own unique self. Any parent of more than one child will easily recognize that each child is uniquely different even though he often grows to look, walk or talk like one of the parents.

By accepting the uniqueness of your baby and responding to his feelings and your own, your child will be provided with the opportunity to develop at his own speed and in his own way. By trying to understand the child as he really is, rather than trying to mould him into our preconceived idea of what he should be, we can provide structure and form within which the child can grow. To understand truly the growth and development of the child we have to be aware of the influences of his environment, his heredity, and his unique self.

Providing the child with a consistent environment, a rhythmic day, and meaningful interactions will allow him to learn to know the world and feel safe in it, and will form an essential basis for further learning.

4. The apprentice

There was a time when in many paths parenting was a much clearer task. It happened without much thought being given to it. When most people lived on farms, they lived with the cycle of the year, learning from the laws of nature. They planted and harvested their garden, co-operating with the seasons and learning about the elements. Their life's work was caring for and nurturing animals and plants. Their survival depended directly on the care they gave their land and their animals. Since their life's work was nurturing and caring for things, they could care for their babies out of the same life-style. They taught their children out of the realities of surviving on a farm. Their way of life provided the opportunity to be aware of the subtle, more slowly changing things in the world. They were able to live with, experience, and know the laws of nature and the great wisdom inherent in nature. They did not have the opportunity of attempting to manipulate nature with clever ideas, but rather tried to understand nature. In their search for understanding they became wise. Since the children were needed to help on the farm, they were taught at an early age how to care for the animals, help with the planting, weeding, harvesting and with food preparation. They learned to milk the cows and churn the butter. They saw barns being built, trees felled, soap being made. What they saw as children was what they did as adults and so they learned how to provide for themselves in this physical world. They knew it and understood it. What they learned, they needed to know.

The world changed and slowly but surely the hard work of the farm life did not have to be followed. There were other choices in the world. You could move to town, earn money, and buy your food and clothes. For a while sons learned their father's trade and so the family's way of life was still a model for the children. The daughters learned how to be wives and learned cooking, canning, sewing, spinning, weaving, knitting and crocheting.

As we look back in history at parenting we find a common theme in the parent-child relationship. The child learned from the parent. The child was apprenticed to the parents to learn how to live in the world. The parent accepted the fact that all the skills for living had to be learned and they taught them to their children. Children grew up learning the skills they needed to provide for themselves in life.

And that is another part of *who* a child is. She is an apprentice to the parent to learn about the world that she lives in. That is *what* parents do. They teach their child about the world. *Why* do they do it? Hopefully to allow the child to learn how to function in the world; so that she can develop her own unique abilities and talents and give them to the world as the gift that she has brought. To allow the world to progress in a more human way. To allow all men to live in freedom, equality and brotherhood. As a parent, how can we do this?

The child has come to us as an apprentice. She looks to us to teach her about the art and science of living in this world. Sadly, the apprenticeship way of learning is slowly disappearing from our life-style. The loss is great because it provided for many important lessons in living. It made it all right not to *know* how to do something. It acknowledged that skills had to be learned from a craftsman and then practiced. It taught caring for, not just using things. It gave heroes to look up to and admire. It showed that being really good at something did matter and that it took time and came from practice. It didn't happen instantly without effort.

When parents intuitively had this apprentice relationship with their children, the parents' task was clearer. It took many hands to run the farm or the family business. It was necessary to have large families to meet the needs of caring for oneself in the world. The children were needed and they knew that; out of being needed they learned the many skills that were required to survive in their world. Later they would use these skills to take care of their own families. The child knew that what she was doing mattered and this gave her a sense of worth. She did not necessarily like what she was doing, but she did know that she mattered and what she did mattered. She learned to be a caring person by looking after the things that her family had worked to acquire, and needed for their work and life-style. She cared for the animals that were so important to them for their food and for the help on the farm. She knew the world and the skills that were so important to meet it. She knew that people mattered and that they were more than animals and more than machines. She didn't just think about it, she lived it.

When families lived in the cycles of nature, not only by a clock and calendar, it was quite easy to understand when the fields had to be cultivated to prepare for planting time, and that sowing the seed had to be completed in the spring of the year. Harvesting had to be done as the fruits, grains, and vegetables ripened. It was not an arbitrary decision to argue about. The framework of their lives was established through the laws of nature. Families understood the changing of the seasons and the necessity of living in harmony with them. It was apparent that there was a time for each task. The families were dependent on the cycles of nature and on each other. They welcomed the sun and the rain. Children were guided to this nature wisdom from an early age. They lived in it. It was a reality for them. They were apprentices to the life of the farm and through this they learned the realities of the world.

The child-as-apprentice, parent-as-teacher role is still the parenting task, but most of the plot and scenery has changed. How do we find a way to understand this relationship in our complicated sophisticated, mechanized, computerized, synthesized world? We can do this by focusing on the basic concept that our task is still to prepare the child to live in the world, by providing an environment in which the child can learn about the world, by being sensitive to the child's needs and abilities and by timing our teaching to coincide with her ability to learn.

Our teaching needs to be adapted to her natural rhythm of learning. We do not help, but rather hinder if we try to teach things out of phase with her development. Our emphasis needs to be on the child's learning, not on our teaching.

It is interesting to observe that baby grows and develops from the head down. We don't try to teach her to sit if she hasn't developed neck control to enable her to support her own head. We don't try to get her to walk until she has developed trunk control and learned to creep and then to crawl. The stages and sequences are extremely important and we don't want to bypass one and leave a gap in her physical development.

This is more apparent in physical development but it also applies to intellectual development. In the first five or six years of the child's life amazing growth and development are going on. This growth is harmonized by physical activity, feelings of security and living and playing imaginatively. It is not an appropriate time for intellectual learning. It is possible, but for what purpose? Is our goal to make parents feel proud and teachers feel clever? At what cost?

We can take a tree and by clipping its roots, by limiting the soil and water we give it, we can create a miniature tree, a bonsai. But what are we really doing, what is our purpose? We prove man can be clever and manipulate nature. That is not our goal in parenting. Rather it is to get to know each child as the unique individual she is, while helping her learn that the world is full of other unique individuals and all people need to be considered. We do not think of her as dumb or smart. We realize that there is a great deal to learn in the world and we try to teach it in such a way that it can be learned.

We are guided by the question, 'Will this behaviour, feeling, action be useful to her in getting along in this world?' We base our decisions on what is right for the child, not what pleases us as the parents, or what pleases the neighbours. We have different answers for different children, for each child is different. Different parents have different answers too, depending on their own values and life styles, but if they are guided by what is right for the child, chances are the decision will be right.

We encourage learning by imitation, learning by discovery. Different things have to be learned in different ways. Learning by discovery provides the child with an opportunity to develop creativity.

Baby is learning all the time. While sitting in her high chair she lets go of her spoon and it falls. She is learning about gravity. She is not a bad girl, she is learning. She will also learn something about you from your reaction to this. What do you want her to know about this way of learning, this learning by discovery? We are back to working out our own philosophy, trying to decide what is important in the world and how we want our child to get to know the world.

Back to the spoon that fell on the floor. Baby looks down and sees the spoon. She is learning about space and gravity. She will also learn about you from your reaction to this. If you ignore her, leave the spoon on the floor, she may not try that again. If you get angry or upset she may feel amazed and pretty important that little her can get that reaction from big you. If you make a game of it, give it back to her a few times, saying 'down' when it is on the floor and 'up' when you give it to her, and then 'all done' or 'no more' before you become annoyed by the game, she will have learned about gravity, the meaning of two words, playing games and, that you know when to quit. She will feel safe knowing that you are in control of the situation, while allowing her to explore. Such games also make us aware of how children love repetition. As they get older we frequently hear, 'do it again'.

The early learning of a small child comes from the parents or from those who are caring for her. These people have a significant influence on the child. Don't think that because she is little it doesn't matter. Every experience we have becomes a part of us. What she learns always matters because it is what she will use to function in the world. In learning it is just as easy to learn what is true as it is to learn misinformation. When we learn what is true, we can put it together with other true things we have learned and slowly come to understand the world. If what we learn is not true, it leads us into confusion. If we look about us, we see that confusion reigns and somehow we have to find our way back to understanding our world.

Some years ago the general information was that the thermostat should be left at 68 to 70 degrees Fahrenheit (20°-21°C) all night because it cost more to raise the temperature in the morning than to maintain the temperature through the night. Now that we are to save energy we are told to set the thermostat low at night or turn it off and have it at 68 degrees only in the daytime. I can learn equally easily that, one, you save gas by maintaining an even temperature day and night, or, two, you save gas by turning it off at night and on in the morning. Both cannot be true. I can memorize the information, but if it isn't true I will not be doing what I think I'm doing and I won't increase my understanding of the world. To understand the world and each other we need to seek for what is true and develop a sense for truth.

What a child learns from us helps build her path through the world. Both what we say and what we do matters. There may be pleasure for some adults in teasing a child or having her do funny things to amuse them, but if we have taken on the task of preparing the child for her future in the world we shall not let her be used for amusement. Nor do we take pleasure in having power over her because we are big and she is small. We use our strength to protect and guide her on her path through life. We will enjoy her, love and care for her.

Babies need to be cared for to survive. Nature has equipped babies with a way of letting us know when they do not feel safe, well and in harmony. That is crying. Crying is an innate, not a learned capacity. Real crying comes when the other world around impinges on us and is overwhelming. Real crying needs to be differentiated from learned crying.

Learned crying is what the child's environment teaches her. How a child uses crying she learns from us. It is from us that the child learns how to behave. It is not inevitable that we teach learned crying, but we may have and it is good to know the difference.

Real crying is a natural means of communication and a way of relieving overwhelming emotions. When the baby cries, we need to try to determine why and change whatever is causing the problem. Real crying should not be ignored. Now for that subtle line of differentiation. Neither should crying become a tool of the child's to manipulate us. If crying is the only way that baby can get our attention or the way she gets what she wants when simpler measures have failed, then we have created a problem. If we say 'no' out of habit, the child pleads, then cries, and we say 'yes', we surely have taught them to persevere, cry, and get what they want.

Crying is an expression as laughing is. It is a purely human capacity, reserved for humans. Animals do not laugh and they do not cry. Crying is not bad, it is a human experience. It can be misused, but it is not inherently bad. Parents have a lot to do with how children use or misuse it.

At this point it will be helpful to know about social learning theory. Briefly stated it is that future behaviour is determined by the response to current behaviour. Now, what does that mean to us as parents? It means that from the way we respond or react to what the child is doing now, she learns something from us for the future. She learns how we feel about what she is doing, and probably how we will react when she does it again. The next time a similar situation arises she will call on this experience to guide her. None of this is at a conscious level. She does not think about it, plan and scheme. But it is the way she learns. So do we.

Let's imagine ourselves in a new job. We walk into the office on the first day, sit down at the desk that we think is ours, and everyone in the office laughs. What will we do? First we will probably wonder why, because we were not intending to be funny. If we don't like being laughed at, and have sufficient courage, we may ask some questions. We probably will not sit there again. If we do like the attention we get from being laughed at, then we will be encouraged to do it again. We have learned that when we sit at this desk, people notice us and laugh.

Behavioural theory is a valuable thing to know and use wisely. Our reaction to the child is what helps her to learn what is acceptable and what is unacceptable. It also teaches her what gets our attention. Through the feelings that we know she has as her own, she will 'read' our response. Social learning theory is not a philosophy, is not a tool to be used or avoided, it is a principle, like a natural law. It is an observable reality like fire burns up or water falls down. We need to be aware of those realities; because whether or not it is our intention, we are teaching the child how to behave through our responses to her. That is why rhythm and consistency are so important for the child. She is learning about the world by the interactions she has with it.

When she is trying something new, think how it will seem the fifth time, and if you don't want it as part of your life say 'no' the first time and mean it.

Meaning it is important, because children learn from our attitude as well as our words. If we say 'no' absent-mindedly, chances are she will do it again to see what we really mean.

Behaviour theory can be misused just as fire can be misused. Here there is a subtle difference in how it is used and it is the subtle things in life that are of vital importance. It can be used in two ways. First, it can be used to control our own behaviour and reaction, knowing that there is a future consequence and the child is learning from what is happening now. Knowing that how we respond to this situation tells our child if what she is doing is okay. We are using this knowledge to control our own behaviour. Secondly, it can also be used to control another person at a subconscious level. By knowing basic needs and intentionally not responding to them, we can control another person's behaviour, assuming they have less sophistication in the theory than we do. We are using this same knowledge to control someone else's behaviour. Ideally, we will choose to act out of self control and self discipline so that we can help the child learn to act in a socially appropriate way. We are then structuring her world so that she can learn about it.

We know that she has physiological needs, that she has feelings and that she needs human interaction. What she needs to learn is how to fulfil her own needs in a constructive way. She needs to learn impulse control, how to wait, to take turns, to consider others. If she lives with people she can imitate, who have those qualities, then her learning will be enhanced. If what she sees in her daily life is consistent with what she is told to do, her world will be easier to imitate and comprehend. She needs to learn what is acceptable in the world and what is not. She will learn what is appropriate from how we act, what we tell her, our reaction to her. She needs form and structure to live in and to learn in. She needs to have clearly defined boundaries for her behaviour. Only then can she feel secure and cared for, then she can learn. Her learning is lived and becomes a reality for her.

One of the most fundamental needs of any person is to be affirmed or acknowledged. The most rewarding way is through approval, acceptance and positive affirmation. If this is not available, a child will misbehave to get some acknowledgement — to assure herself that she does exist for herself and for others. Disregarding a child can lead to serious mental health problems.

When the child is doing something that we object to, we need to tell her what to do, not just 'no'. If she is writing on walls, or books or furniture, we give her paper to write on. We tell her that paper is what we write on, not other things. If she is playing with water, splashing and spilling it, we direct her to watering the plants, or washing dishes, or washing the bathtub. We don't stop the activity, but redirect it to where it is appropriate. She has to learn *what to do* and *where to do it*. She does not learn this through 'no'. She learns it by being directed to the appropriate way of doing it. Activity is synonymous with childhood, and we want to direct the activity, not try to stop it. It is almost inevitable that children experiment with anti-social behaviour.

One of their early experiments, frequently around three or four, is spitting. Why remains a mystery to me, but occur it does. When this happens we can simply and firmly say, 'when you need to spit, spit in the toilet.' As we are saying this we carry the child to the bathroom. We stay with her and direct her to spit in the toilet as many times as she wants to. Each time she spits, we respond in the same way. She will learn that there are limits on behaviour, and we will establish those limits.

Biting is frequently the next problem. This can be handled by putting your hand under her lower jaw and quickly closing her mouth when she is about to bite. At the same time say, 'no, biting hurts.' You might add, 'if you need something to bite I will get you a carrot or an apple.' Something that requires using her teeth in an acceptable way.

We do need to establish a guideline for 'no' and there is a fairly simple one. We always say 'no' if what the child is doing will hurt her, hurt another person or damage something. This needs to be consistent and forever. Being destructive to herself, others or things is never all right. If we save our 'no' for these occasions, it will become clear to her what 'no' relates to. Our aim is to make our outer direction become an inner direction. For this to happen there has to be clarity and a pattern to internalize. She needs to realize that being destructive is not all right. If her life is full of 'no' she will feel thwarted, but she will not know what 'no' relates to. It will not be clear to her. If we limit our 'no' to when she is being destructive and guide her to appropriate activities we will be helping her find her way into the world in a constructive way. She needs to get clear messages. Certainly there are times when what the child wants to do is not convenient for others in the family, and this will also be a 'no' or a postponed 'yes'. That is also important for the child to learn: others' needs also have to be considered and we can't always do what we want to do. This is another important part of learning.

Involved explanations and philosophizing are lost on a small child. They don't need to have things made complicated. The world seems complicated enough to them. They need it sorted out, differentiated, and simplified; so that they can understand it. They need to know if what they are doing at the moment is okay or not.

What you will do with Aunt Maude's antique vase is up to you. We need to remember that activity is a natural healthy part of childhood. Babies' most natural way to learn is through exploration. Their sense organs are not so differentiated to them and exploring means seeing, touching, tasting and smelling all at the same time. When they see something they reach for it and put it in their mouth. This is the normal way for them to learn when they are toddlers. As they grow older and their senses are more differentiated then we can tell them to 'just look with your eyes', but that is not possible for a toddler. It will be up to you to decide if Aunt Maude's antique vase is how you want to use your 'no', or if you want to put it away for a while.

A common concept of learning theory is that you

ignore your child when she cries, only give her attention when she is smiling, and then she will grow up
to be a happy and smiling person. By using (or mis-
using) behaviour theory, she is supposed to learn that
her basic need of affirmation will be met only when
she smiles and is happy. The result is supposed to be
a happy, smiling child. Because this is so generally
accepted, it seems important to take a closer look at
the facts. When the baby cries, it is to tell us that
something is wrong. She doesn't feel protected and
safe. The world is overwhelming her. If we ignore
her, what does she learn from this experience? Her
feelings of separateness are confirmed, her vulnera-
bility to the world is confirmed. The world *is* overwhelming. She is unable to do anything about her
discomfort. There is no one to help her or take care
of her. No one comes. She may cry herself to sleep or
eventually stop crying, but what does she learn? She
tucks that sad experience into her storehouse of experiences and if there are enough such experiences
she views the world as an unfriendly place. There is
no basis for security and trust. Her call for help has
not been heeded.

It is probable that this will reduce the child's
crying, because if no one ever comes when she cries,
she may give up this natural resource. She may just
endure. Be aware that extinguishing crying cannot be
equated with a happy child. A truly happy child is
one who is secure and knows that there is someone to
care for her when she needs to be cared for. A happy
child is one who is tuned into her own feelings of
bodily comfort, discomfort and well-being, one who

can trust nature's signals and her feelings, one who is in touch with herself.

If the child is crying because we taught her to, then that is a very different problem. It is still our problem, but the solution will be different. Using behaviour theory with learned behaviour is a very different thing from using it with natural instinctive behaviour. Also remember that behaviour theory can be used two ways: to be conscious of our own behaviour or to manipulate others' behaviour.

If we have taught our child to cry and it is learned crying, then we need to change our responses. It is encouraging to know that if the behaviour that is inappropriate has been learned then a new behaviour can be learned to replace it. Anything that is learned can be unlearned or relearned.

To change behaviour we need to be aware of what happens before the crying and after the crying. We look at what we are doing to encourage it or require it or reward it. Remember, we are talking about learned crying.

We also need to think a bit about the goal of shaping our child into a happy, smiling child. It appears that inevitably means a happy child is one who suppresses her own feelings to meet our expectations or demands. Is that what the world needs to solve the gigantic problems that we are faced with? A world full of happy smiling people who are out of touch with themselves and the reality that is going on around them? Not really. Rather, we need people who are real. People who have the inner ability to find what is true, to sort out the good from the bad and to have the courage to defend what is right and to fight what is wrong. To smile when they feel good and to frown when they don't. It is the inner being of the child that we need to consider, not only the outer countenance. We want to help our child to be robust, yet sensitive: to have a healthy body, to develop feelings that will lead to understanding, and a mind that can search for truth and reality.

What is in the child's environment will become internalized by him. The formed and consistent environment will become an inner structure. The care she has been given will become an inner caring. As she becomes an adult, what she has internalized from her environment, she will be able to put back into the world in a heightened way. If she has had the opportunity to experience the attitude of devotion, a reverence for nature, mutual respect and morality, she will have the opportunity to develop her own capacities for love and wisdom.

5. Learning about the world

The child is born with her own innate qualities and talents and her own individual temperament, but she must learn an enormous amount about the world in order to be able to function in it. The more complex the world becomes the more there is to learn about. Each of us has learned so much within a lifetime, it is staggering to contemplate. The baby must learn how to communicate her bodily needs so that she can be cared for, she must learn to understand and speak the language of her family, she must learn the non-verbal as well as the verbal language, she must learn to recognize people and objects, to identify smells and tastes, to sit, to crawl, to walk, to speak, to think, to play, to work. The parents' influence in all this learning is immense. As we sort out who the child is, from what she has to learn about the world, we will slowly understand what we must teach her.

The child has her own feelings. When her bodily needs are met and they function in harmony, she feels comfort and that gives her pleasure. Her own inner wisdom tells her that harmony is health-giving, life-giving and the biological state to strive for. Just as a plant that is given too much or not enough water, sunlight or food loses its vitality and dies; baby too has basic physiological needs to be met. The flower has no brain and nervous system to summon us when it is out of balance, but baby does. Our baby can signal us when the balance is upset and harmony is replaced by disharmony. She will fuss and cry. When we find the appropriate rhythm for baby's care, then we can maintain this physiological harmony.

When the harmony is lost, when the physiological needs of warmth and food and liquid are not met, then she experiences discomfort. Her inner wisdom tells her this is not the health-giving state and she calls to us for help. She cannot meet her own needs, so she signals to us to care for her.

How we respond is the beginning of her learning about the world. She learns that she is separate and that the world comes to meet her and goes away. That is not a pleasant experience for a helpless little one with feelings. How unpleasant will be determined by the baby's individual temperament, sensitivity and physiology. Some children will tolerate the separation as long as their own basic needs of food, warmth and liquids are regularly met, other children will feel desperate. How we care for our baby's needs is guided by what baby tells us. It will be an interaction between parents and child, not an implementation of absolute rules blindly followed.

Baby's first learning is a more global social interaction between her physiological needs and the important people who meet her needs. As she becomes more awake and alert we can observe the beginnings of her discrimination. She follows with her eyes, she seems to listen, she enjoys her parents softly singing to her, she looks at her hands, learns to move them and eventually brings them together to touch and clasp. She is also learning to vocalize, and babble in preparation for learning to repeat sounds that she has heard often enough for them to be familiar.

Baby is learning control of her body: the overcoming of her reflexes and orientation in space from the wisdom of nature. She is developing her inner organs and their functions out of the wisdom of nature. These are immensely important tasks.

Baby learns not only from the wisdom of nature, but also from her parents. What baby first learns from her parents she learns through imitation. Imitation is a natural response of the child and it is her earliest way of learning from her environment. We say 'bye-bye' and wave to the child. We do this many times and then the baby learns to wave bye-bye. By doing the same thing several times, the child learns to recognize it and imitate it. First we wave when she waves, next she associates the word 'bye' with waving, finally she learns to wave when we say 'bye'.

Children are not the only ones who learn from imitation. Suppose we as adults decide to learn a new language. What do we ask of our teacher? First we hope that the teacher realizes we don't know the language and that he will be patient with our attempts to learn. When the teacher speaks to us in this unknown language it will be a combination of bewildering sounds. We probably won't be able to pick out any words unless one is repeated frequently enough for us to begin to recognize it. It may become a familiar sound, but we still won't know what it means or what it refers to. If we hear it often though, it will become familiar and then we will be able to learn to say it. After we say it a few times we will be able to remember it, but we will still have to learn what it means or describes.

Baby has this same task in learning our language; learning the sounds, how they go together in words, remembering the words and associating them with what they describe. An amazing process.

We can discover that speech is not an innate quality that spontaneously evolves by realizing that babies speak the language of their parents. They speak the language that they hear in their environment. Babies of English parents speak English, French babies speak French, Chinese babies speak Chinese, babies in the southern United States have southern accents, in eastern United States they have eastern accents. The baby needs to hear the language spoken to be able to learn the language of her parents. She does innately have the ability to make sounds, but does not know how to form them into our words. This she must learn from us. To learn our language, she must hear our language. By hearing familiar words, she will begin to imitate their sounds. Dada, mama, bye, become familiar words that she will attempt to imitate. She will be exceedingly pleased when she is able to form our words and become more a part of our world. Parents talking to a baby is vitally important. It acknowledges her, it includes her in our world and it lets her hear the sound of our words, our language; so she can learn it.

Imitation is one way to learn and that is the way

baby will learn to talk. Discovery is another way to learn. She hits the bath water with her hand and it splashes her in the face. She is surprised. If it splashes mother too, and mother gets angry, baby will have made two discoveries and may have trouble deciding what discovery to respond to.

As we grow in our awareness as parents we discover the seemingly paradoxical fact that what we help the child to become as an adult is not what we expect of her as a child. A child is not a miniature adult. For her to be friendly and at ease with people as an adult does not mean that we expose her to a great variety of people as an infant. Rather it is necessary that first she have the opposite experience: to be cared for and protected by her parents, or her special few, and out of the space of protection and safety she may then develop the qualities of trust and confidence. Friendliness comes from this inner trust, knowing oneself well enough to feel safe in reaching out to know another.

It is amazingly easy to fall into the trap of telling a child, 'quit acting like a child!' Forgetting that is precisely what she is supposed to be doing. A child by nature is not intended to be treated like a miniature adult. The years of childhood are precious few, and each of us has only one chance in this life to be a baby, an infant, a toddler, pre-schooler. We have the rest of our lives to be adults; so we need to let children be children. Let them use this time to live in their imagination and develop it to discover the world, to feel and touch. Then we will have mature adults.

Our grandparents had some philosophies about

children that have gone out of style, and probably rightly so. For example, 'Children should be seen and not heard.' The content may not have been appropriate, but it shows us that they did realize a child was different from an adult. Because of their life style it was more apparent that you 'can't expect a boy to do a man's work'. When you are all working together for survival, you have a better basis for determining who can do what. That is past. We no longer have those experiences to help us observe as clearly what a child's ability, limitations and true nature are.

Another old adage was 'spare the rod and spoil the child'; and we also need to look at that. It sounds like spoiling equates to being too nice. When we say she's spoiled, what do we mean? What spoils a child?

First let us try to understand what spoiling is. When we say we spoil the soup, or spoil the picture, or spoil the story, we mean we have injured it or damaged it. Something that is spoiled is damaged and so it is with children. If a child is spoiled she is damaged or injured. She hasn't learned about the world and how to live in it. We don't spoil a child when we are caring people helping the child to learn about the world and her place in it. We cannot spoil a child by attending to her physiological, biological, or emotional needs. We can spoil a child, damage a child, if we don't help her learn self-discipline, self-control and consideration for others.

Now we are free of the parenting traditions of our grandparents and free of the life that made us so dependent on, but also aware of, the laws of nature. In general, we have left behind the authoritarian approach to parenting. In fact, the expectation of absolute obedience has gone to the opposite extreme of permissiveness: from one extreme to another. With the other extreme we face the problems inherent in that. If the child does not have the defined limits she needs on her path, she gets lost in the world jungle. Permissive parents find themselves in impossible situations for themselves and their children. Family living does not exist, is not possible, when each person is doing as he pleases. What pleases one person may conflict with what pleases another. Permissiveness bewilders the child or turns her into a despot. Neither is a useful role for living in the world.

Now that we are free of the strong traditions that built a framework for family life, and we are no longer dependent on the laws of nature for our framework, where will our direction come from? How can we find the guidance we need to help our children grow up to be responsible citizens in a world that will probably become even more complex than the one we are living in now, a world that we can't even visualize or predict?

It is clear that it is no longer enough only to teach current appropriate social behaviour, because society is changing too rapidly. The child will need to have lived with reasonable discipline so that she can have gained self-discipline. Please note, not punishment, discipline.

Inevitably any child will at some time transgress the rule of no destruction to others, himself or things. How that is handled will depend on you, the child, and the situation. If some discipline is indicated it is important that it be a natural consequence to remedy the destruction. If a window has been broken, then money can be saved from her allowance to pay for replacement. Having her help in cleaning up and replacing the window will also be important. She will then learn why breaking a window is unacceptable. If she hurts a friend, then she can be restricted from playing with the friend. It will help her learn about the world and the importance of self control and self discipline.

Punishment takes on a very different character and it involves inflicting some kind of pain. For a young child we may use a light tap to get her attention if she persists when we say no, but it will not be sufficient to cause pain. Realizing that what is in her outer world becomes an inner trait we will understand that we want to help the child develop self discipline, not self punishment.

What a child learns from her parents is what she will use for meeting life and the world. The child puts her trust in her parents to guide her through this complex world. She trusts the parents will have the wisdom to say 'yes' or 'no' when it is needed. There are many things the child, as apprentice, must learn about the world to meet its conflicting expectations and demands. We can teach her no longer only about the work on our farm and the rules of our village, but about the whole world and how to meet it. It is an awesome responsibility to know about the whole earth and even the cosmic world beyond; to live out of a sense of responsibility amidst many choices, no longer out of necessity, to learn to care for all people, to be responsible for herself, to be reasonable, to allow others to be themselves, to develop their own sense of values, to find truth and reality, to work, and play, and enjoy life. All these things matter.

Parents no longer have children because they need them to help do the work on the farm. Parents now, generally, have children because they want them and feel it is a natural way to live. Sometimes, of course, it just happens. The parents who want the child and prepare for her arrival may be surprised to find how complex it has all become. They want to be good parents, whatever that is, and do the right thing, whatever that is. What is that in our world of endless choices, in a world where we are not as pressed by natural needs, where we have the possibility of choosing what we want to do and how to do it? How can we be good parents and prepare our children for an ever faster changing world where reality and illusion are so intertwined that we look at a plant and can't tell if it is real or plastic, a world where so much of the natural world is imitated, an inert world that does not communicate with us? We cannot learn anything about the nature of a rose from a plastic one, even though they look alike. This natural way of learning is no longer inherently there.

Somehow we have to find it again. The child still needs to know about the world of nature. She lives in that as well as in the mechanized and synthesized world.

What do we do about chores for children? Why has that become a problem? Where once a child was needed to do a part of the work that had to be done, now it is less so. We may feel as parents that we have too many tasks. It may be irritating to see strong healthy young people idle, while they are wondering what to do with their time, complaining about not having anything to do. Somehow it seems right to expect them to do something in return for what is provided for them in the home. Behind these vague feelings there is a reality.

Each of us takes a great deal from the world. We are dependent in many ways on others. The food we eat, the clothes we wear, the homes we live in, the cars we ride in, all come from the gifts of nature and the efforts of our fellow men. Because we pay money for things that may somehow give us the idea we deserve them, that possessing them is our right. But we could have all the money in the world and not be able to use it if others stopped their work. If all the manufacturers of materials decided to stop weaving cloth, where would we be? We can't make clothes out of money.

At some level of consciousness we know how dependent we are on the natural world and others. One of the basic needs of man is to feel that he is contributing something back to the world that provides for him. We are not talking about economics or money, we are talking about human deeds. Each of us needs to contribute to the world, to do something in the world. Without this opportunity we become detached from the world. It is very uncomfortable always to be receiving and never giving or returning. It strips us of our human dignity and offends our subconscious knowledge that we can be creative and productive.

This is not always apparent in children and their behaviour may indicate they object to doing tasks at home. This resistance on the child's part comes in part from an uncertainty that we are right in our expectations. We may have a vague sense of guilt when we do not understand what is right, when, and why. By thinking of our child as an apprentice, on a path through childhood, we can find our way to this reality. It is not only because we need the job done, that is not the only consideration. It is also because the child needs to learn to function in the world. As the child grows, she needs the opportunity to learn skills that she will be expected to have as an adult. She needs to learn to care for things, repair things, and make things. She needs to know how to wash clothes, fold clothes, put them in their proper place, iron clothes, grow food, prepare food, serve food, wash dishes, dust, sweep, cut the grass, take responsibility for pets. There is a great deal to know in the world. The more of these skills a person has, the more she can feel at home in the world.

As we realize this, then we will see the need of varying the tasks of the child. If we assign tasks only on the basis that we need them done, then we are not thinking of the child in the same way. Generally, the child's help is not so vitally significant. How often we think, 'it would be easier to do it myself, and quicker too'. True as that may be, that is not the point. Even though teaching a new skill is more time-consuming than doing it ourselves the child's learning about the world is of primary importance. We could manage ourselves, but that is only part of the reality. It is still true that what we know, we have learned, somehow, from someone or by discovery. All tasks, including washing, ironing, gardening, maintenance have to be learned.

Have you noticed what the number one job is for boys at least in suburban neighbourhoods? Yes, taking out the trash. Frequently that is the only job that they have for months on end. For the girls, it is doing the dishes. In general it is not because we are planning to prepare them for these two tasks in life. As a matter of fact, we couldn't employ that many rubbish men or dish washers. It is because at some level of consciousness we know the children 'should' be doing something around the house, but we are nor clear why or what.

As we become aware of this basis for helping, then we see the need for varying the tasks of the child. We don't meet her need to learn about life if we limit her to one task. We only make her resent helping in most cases. The child is aware that her help is not so necessary to the functioning of the family. She knows the parents could manage without her, and perhaps more efficiently. It is not like it was on the farm, not for the child or for the parents. Children do still need to learn how to do things and how to care for things. When the parent is aware that the child needs instruction to learn about the world, that all things must be learned, then practiced, then done independently, he will see that the child has the opportunity to learn a variety of skills to help her gain a feeling of self-dependence in the world. The more we know about the things around us, how to care for them, how to fix them and how to make them, the more we feel at home in the world.

It will be a very different experience for the child, if our approach to her comes from helping her to learn about the world, to learn skills, and to learn how to work together.

6. The golden mean

As we go through life with our apprentice, we find what an awesome task it is. He needs to learn about the world as it is today, to have some knowledge of the world past, and to be allowed to dream for the future. There are different things to learn from other parts of the world. Countries have different customs, values, and priorities, as well as different climates, vegetation and animals. There is much to learn. The world is full of variation; the intermixing and inter-workings of substances and influences. We can observe the effects of the varying combinations of influences.

The same variety of plant appears differently in different locations and will certainly look different at various times. A child observing a dandelion might tell us it has a yellow flower, another child observing another dandelion might say 'no', it has a fluffy white ball that floats away when you blow on it. Plants change in time. Plants also change according to the location. We can observe the way a dandelion grows when it has ample sunshine and ample water; we then compare it with a dandelion that grows in the shade, but with ample water; again we compare one that grows in ample sunshine, but with limited water. We can observe how the dandelion changes according to the elements available in its environment. Out of our own observation we can see how they vary, depending on the amount of sunshine and water that they get. Certainly, any time we look at the plant we are looking at a dandelion, growing within the constraints of the basic dandelion form, but with variations of height, and density, depending on its growth cycle, the life phase, and environment. There may be no flower, a yellow flower, or a soft white puff, it may be compact or rangy. It is different at different times, and different places, but it is still a dandelion.

We don't know all about a dandelion if we have only seen one in one place. If we pull it from the ground and take it into a classroom, we are not really learning about a dandelion. To know it and understand it, we have to watch it in the earth, and observe it over time in the world that influences it.

We may value it, or we may object to its presence. Some people put the dandelion greens in their salad or steam them for a vegetable. Some people grow them by the acre to be used in chicken feed, some people make wine from them, and some people pull them out of their lawn while grumbling about them. We cannot think of them as good or bad, but we can think of them as varied.

Children vary too, only more so. They differ from one another, but they also are different at different times, and they are also affected by their environment. They interact with it and they are influenced by it. In their lives they may grow, and blossom, and eventually become fruitful if they are nurtured by their environment.

Each child has a basic inherited form, conditioned

by his inheritance from his parents. He lives in his own environmental influences and he also has his own unique individuality. All aspects are observable. We accept that each child will be different, that there will be variations and yet there will also be things in common. We have our human nature in common. All children need adequate and appropriate food, clothing and shelter. They need to be affirmed and acknowledged. All need structure and form surrounding them. All need loving care. All children start out their lives eager to learn about the world, they laugh when they are happy and cry when they are sad. These are parts of human nature.

It is this human nature that we want to encourage and direct and understand to help the child find his way into the world in a balanced way. This nature includes our feelings, our thoughts, our activity and our human individuality.

We have discovered that with our human form we are able to be active in a unique way. We do many different things. Our limbs are differentiated, our legs and feet are very different from our arms and hands. This gives us an endless variety of possible activities. We have also found that we have the ability to get to know our environment and ourselves through our feelings, and we can express our feelings through our arms and our legs. We can do this in music, dance, painting, modelling, in general through the arts and through movement. We can express our feelings. We can also kiss and hug, we can shake hands and express our feelings by using our limbs in another way. We can act the way we feel.

Something else is true about our feelings. We can change them by the way we act or by what we do. We can dispel a feeling of sadness by putting on a favourite lively tune. If we feel nervous and hassled, we can change that to a feeling of calm, perhaps through knitting or crocheting, embroidery or wood-working. By engaging in an artistic activity in a creative way, we can create a different feeling. We can learn about the world through our feelings, and we can create new feelings.

We also have our thinking. Thinking also affects our feelings and feelings accompany thoughts. We open the mail box and find a package. We think it is for us and we feel excited. We think a friend who is away has sent us a special treat. We feel warmly toward that friend. We open the box and we are delighted to find that what we thought was true; and we feel good. Or perhaps, when we open the box we find it it is really for someone else and then we feel disappointed. In both cases our first feelings are consequences of our thoughts. The feelings changed as we sorted out the reality of the situation, but nevertheless the feeling was first associated with a thought. We can sit and day-dream without any precipitating cause and experience a variety of feelings. We can imagine that we are famous, respected, the centre of attention. We feel important, pleased, or wise. We can think we are neglected, unimportant, unappreciated, then we feel glum. Feelings are part of us and our feelings change. They can also be created and they can be changed.

Thoughts are also there. Some thoughts seem to

parade through our minds with little or no direction from us. Other times thoughts follow the direction that we choose. We can concentrate our thoughts on a particular subject and consciously combine ideas. We can think about what we do, about what we observe, and about how we feel. We can also think about thinking. We can wonder if what we are thinking about or what we have been told is true. We can think, we can feel and we can do things: each is separate and yet they are related parts of us. It is the content and relationship of our thinking, feeling and doing that forms our personality.

We can think of feeling, thinking and doing as three horses pulling a cart. When they work together, in harmony, the journey is smooth. As adults we can add another ingredient. We can become the driver of those three horses. By using our ego, or individuality, we can be in control of the harmony and balance of our thinking, feeling and doing. Then we can act out of a reasoned decision rather than reacting to our life's journey. As adults we can learn to direct these aspects of ourselves, as the driver of the cart directs the horses. However, this is not possible in the same way for the child. He needs his family to provide a harmonious environment with outer direction and constraints for him.

We serve the child best when we acknowledge all parts of his personality, nourish them, so that they can develop and then help him balance and harmonize them. We recognize this when we see the child is getting too boisterous and his feelings are carrying him away in his activity. We tell him 'that is enough', 'calm down'. This is also an important part of learning about himself and the world: acknowledging and allowing for all facets of him while creating for him the boundaries of the path. By providing for experiences for his feelings, his activities, and later his thinking in an enriching way, we allow him the opportunity to get to know himself and the world.

The toddler is always on the go, living in his experience of activity. He learns easily by imitating what we do. He learns most naturally through doing. He loves doing what we do. This is the natural way for a young child to learn. Not through intellectual directions or admonishments, but by learning through his activity. By accepting this way of learning and providing him with good models to imitate, we learn how to work with a child of this age. When we want him to change an activity, we join him in his world and then we let him imitate us.

If he is playing with his trucks, we join him, and we tell the truck driver we are going to drive into the bathroom and tell Mr Duck that it is time to fill the tub so that Mr Duck can go swimming. Then his world moves on in a harmonious way and he isn't wrenched from his world of play. We live in his world with him. We structure this world for him and then we are building a natural relationship with him at this age. Take note that we are not letting him do what he wants when he wants to, but we are directing his world from his perspective. We lead him through his day by providing the form and structure for him to imitate. At this age, he is eager to learn about the world and he is inquisitive. We want to keep those qualities alive in him; so that he will be able to approach the world with an open inquiring mind, with a love of discovery and learning. Be aware of these natural qualities in your child and appreciate them. Also direct them, show him what to do and where to do it.

If the child has been cared for and allowed to develop in his own way in the appropriately structured and balanced environment he will have a good start to becoming a well-balanced person and we shall not have to worry about him becoming one-sided. This is rather a pitfall of adults, especially in our world that seems to value thinking and cleverness above all else. However, if we ask the child to be intellectual and clever, he will try to give us what we ask for and we are building in a problem. Being clever is very different from being wise and understanding.

We want to allow the child to develop in a natural way, neither forcing nor retarding him, providing him with the experiences that are appropriate for his age in a harmonious structured way.

Techniques for teaching reading at an early age have been developed. It is important to ask, what is the advantage of a child reading at three or four? Some children can be trained to do this. It is possible, but is it right? Is it the natural sequence of development? If he first has the opportunity to learn to move with ease, to discover the world, to develop his muscles, his co-ordination and his balance, and to allow his nervous system to mature, he is equipped in later life with a body that has developed naturally. With the current concern over poor reading at the high school level, it is quite remarkable that we haven't stopped to take a look at what we are doing and tried to assess it. While reading is being taught at an earlier age and as young children have been asked to sit passively and quietly in the classroom, reading skills have declined in general. Perhaps it is time to go back and allow young children to explore, discover, play games, discover rhythm, and enjoy their early childhood until it is time for first grade.

Having a child who reads at an early age may please the teacher, because she has been able to teach the child and it may make the parents proud of having produced this clever tot, but what we are looking for is rather what is right for the child. What will serve him best as he prepares for his life?

We want to give the child the opportunity to experience all of his qualities: his thinking of course, but also his feelings, and his ability to move and to do things. All these qualities need to be nurtured in childhood; so that they can be educated for adulthood. We want to make it possible for the child eventually to grow to the point where as an adult it will be possible to act out of an inner harmony of these three aspects of himself. What is present in the environment of the child will be internalized by him, it will become part of his life's experience and later will be a part of his personality.

If he has had the experience of harmony and balance in his environment as a child, he will later have an inner knowledge of the experience of balance and harmony. He will then have a head start toward becoming a harmoniously functioning, balanced adult.

A balanced person is healthy, both mentally and physically. When a person can direct his own feelings, his thinking, and his activity in harmony he has the basis for directing his life, rather than being a victim of life. He will be able to act in life rather than react. Again we shall not expect the child to have the qualities that we expect of ourselves, just as we don't expect the seedling in our garden to bear fruit already. Childhood is the child's time to be a child, not a miniature adult; a time to be nourished and cared for, protected and guided with love and understanding. He needs the chance to unfold and develop his capacities before they can be harmonized and balanced. He needs the opportunity to discover himself, all aspects of himself. Then these qualities can eventually grow to the point where as an adult it will be possible to develop inner direction and self-control.

We allow the child to be a child and unfold his natural capacities so that as an adult he will have the three aspects of his personality available to work with, and to mould into an instrument that will serve him well in his life. He will know himself as a feeling, thinking and doing person, one who can direct these natural qualities in himself. By providing a balanced harmonious environment, we help the child grow in harmony and it is in harmony that we have the basis for true morality. Not a morality based on local ideas or rules, but a fundamental universal morality. A morality that is based on balance, a balance between two extremes, neither too much nor too little.

What is a morality based on balance? Let us look at the quality of courage. What is courage and where does it come from? It is a quality that is needed in any environment and at first may seem difficult to explain. Frequently it is thought of as a virtue that is the opposite of cowardice, but that does not tell us what it is, rather it tells what it is not, giving us only partial understanding.

Courage is the balance between cowardice and foolhardiness. It is midway between two extremes. It is not courageous to run headlong into a destructive situation or to do something that is flagrantly dangerous. That is foolhardy. Virtue comes from going to neither extreme: neither withdrawing out of cowardice nor acting out of foolhardiness, neither succumbing to self-seeking nor to self-annihilation, rather standing upright between the temptation on each side. In courage we stand balanced, knowing both extremes, and choosing a harmonious blending of the two.

We act in a courageous way when we stand in a clear and thoughtful way for what we know is right. We neither run from the situation nor sacrifice ourself to it. We use reason and balance, and then we have a morality based on acting out of harmony and balance.

Another important quality to nurture is an interest in the world. It is our interest in the people around us that leads us to care for others, to be concerned for others. Without interest in the world around us, we become apathetic and then what goes on around us does not matter to us. What happens in the world and to other people in the world does matter. We need to be aware of what is wrong and what is right.

We do not necessarily have to condemn or condone, we do not need to judge, but we do need to be aware and to evaluate. When something destructive is done, it is wrong, and an awareness of that is important.

When we are trusting and accepting of everything and tolerate corruption and evil we have become apathetic. We adopt the attitude, perhaps subconsciously, that it is not our problem and it does not matter. It is certainly possible that it is something beyond our control, that we cannot intervene, but it is still essential that we are clear within ourselves that it is destructive and not moral.

It is possible to err in the other extreme from apathy to fanaticism, to fanaticism fired by curiosity. Then our own importance and ideas become exaggerated and we take on a 'cause' without true understanding of the problems. We are reacting out of our own feelings and are not really relating to the problem that exists. When we become fanatic, we are on a separate course from our fellow man, one that can lead to self-destruction or annihilation. Neither fanaticism nor apathy serves us well in the world but interest does.

By being interested in the world around us, we come to care for the world. We do not think only of ourselves and of gratifying our own immediate needs. We think of ourselves in relation to the whole world, the world of our fellow man, of nature, of the eternal aspects of life. Through feelings of interest we connect ourselves with the world in a caring way. It is through feelings of interest and caring that we are able to love.

By caring enough about a person to let him be

himself, we learn to love. We care for him as he is and dream with him that he will be able to unfold his real human qualities. We inwardly experience the other person.

We are again in the realm of important subtleties. We experience the other person in ourselves — we do not experience ourselves in the other person. We allow him to be. We do not try to dominate, control, or seduce him. Neither do we obliterate ourselves and serve his needs and desires and forsake our own. We stand in the balance, upright. We allow ourselves to be and we allow the other to be. *I* and *thou*. We take responsibility for ourselves and we allow the other person to take responsibility for himself, not as a child of course, but when he becomes an adult. Becoming responsible is a gradual learning process and not something that magically happens at eighteen or twenty-one. However, it is the ultimate goal for the child for whom we are now responsible.

For young children, we provide a place of love and balance and morality for them to live in. As they grow they first imitate this in their play and later in their friendships. As they mature, we give them opportunities to be responsible. We help them to find their balance and stand upright. When they are being tempted in either direction we help them to know when to say 'yes' and when to say 'no'. We allow them to experience morality, to imitate it, to develop it in themselves and eventually to try it in the world.

As we reaffirm the wisdom of the ancient sages about the golden mean, we learn that morality in life is not either/or. Good is not the opposite of bad: good is the balance between two extremes.

This has very practical applications in our world. When we realize that working a twelve-hour day is not right, we don't go to the opposite extreme and think life without work is the desired state. For meaningful living we need to care about and be involved in the world. Excess in either direction leads to distortion of living. When a person is not involved in meaningful activity, he feels estranged from the world, unable to contribute to it and participate in it. He loses interest and becomes apathetic. When a person has too much work to do, he may become obsessed with his own task and may lose the perspective of others in the world. He can become so involved in what he is doing that he is unable to stand back and take a look at his work in relationship to the world and to others in the world. It is important to take time to contemplate what we are doing and how we are doing it.

We need the balance of working at a meaningful task, a time for artistic creativity, and a time for observation and introspection. We need to be in the world and we need to withdraw into ourselves, just as we need to inhale and exhale.

The concept of balance and moderation encounters more resistance when we get into the realm of economics. Recognizing that money is an arbitrary, man-created means of exchange, it is difficult to conceive that there is not enough money in the world to allow all men to live in dignity. It is not so difficult to see that money is inadequately and unequally distributed. We shall not consider the having too much or too little aspect of money, but possible relationships to money.

One extreme is the person who puts money as the primary value in the world and uses it as a gauge to assess the value or importance of people and possessions. The more it costs, the better it is or the more money the person has, the better he is. The primary focus is on the money and acquiring it. Money is valued for its own sake, not as a means of exchange. The person spends money as part of his identity, and uses possessions in the same way.

The other extreme is the person who is very frugal and won't spend money on necessary items. He saves things he has no use for to avoid having to spend money at a later time, just in case. He avoids spending money if at all possible, and may take it to the extreme of avoiding earning money. Despite his intentions to discredit the importance of money he has fallen into the trap of materialism too. His primary motives also relate to money. He too is in the grip of materialism, in the opposite extreme.

The reality is that we all need material things to live in the world. We all need clothes, shelter, and food. In general we cannot each provide all of these needs for ourselves. We depend on others to provide some of these things for us. Whether we barter or purchase, the fact remains that part of our needs and possessions come from someone else. In modern society we do need money to buy these things. The real value, however, is in the items needed, not in the money required to buy them.

We need some way to acquire the items necessary for survival. There are a variety of ways to carve out the portion of the world that we need to sustain our physical needs. Somehow these things have to be provided for; for ourselves and our children. The quantity and quality of what we each feel we need will vary, but within that wide range somehow we have to obtain what we need to survive. It is not the only important consideration in the world, but if our basic physical survival needs cannot be met, there is little energy for more enhancing activity. We have to take a small part of the world and make it ours.

Hopefully we are doing this as a free deed without any expectation of appreciation. The expectation is a deadly trap. We shall always be disappointed. The general reality is that another person cannot know what was involved in what we did. They won't know how long it took or how hard it was. Chances are they won't want to hear about it either. Don't sacrifice yourself to others, they don't want it and they don't want to hear about it. It is much better to give only what you can give freely without expecting gratitude or appreciation in return. Do things because you think they need to be done and you want to do them. Work together with mutual respect and a sharing of tasks. This is a goal worth striving for and an important quality for your child to learn.

When things are done out of the need of the task, without bringing in other reasons, we have made a giant step toward living a fulfilling life. You wash and wax the floor because it needs to be cared for, you cut the grass because it needs to be cared for. Doing either job to please someone else or to have them appreciate you, deprives you of the satisfaction of a job well done which cannot come to you in any other way. The focus is not on your performance, but the focus is on the job that has been done. It is visible and rewarding. You feel good about the results and your deed; you don't need someone to tell you that you are good.

As children grow into their adult responsibilities, they will be very fortunate if they have learned to do jobs well and look at what they have done with a sense of satisfaction. When we know how to care for ourselves in the world we do not need to resort to the undignified process of manipulation. Manipulation is only necessary when you can't do something that you need or want done. Then you have to cleverly scheme to bring about through someone else what you want. Going through life manipulating others to do what you want is a very unrewarding way to live. By helping our apprentice learn how to function in the world, to develop practical skills, and to care for things, he will not have to be a manipulator or a self-sacrificer. He will approach life with the knowledge that he can manage.

By learning about the world in a balanced and harmonized way and using that harmony to unfold his talents and skills, he will be able to function in the world as it is today and dream about a tomorrow that can be better.

7. Personal space

Most often when we think of space, we think of a measurable physical space. Is the space big enough to park the car? Is there enough space for a bigger refrigerator? It is easily and clearly definable. We also have the concept of outer space which is less easily defined, but still measurable and definable by astronomers and aerospace engineers.

Each person occupies a space which is in part measurable by their size. How much physical space a person occupies depends on his height and weight and bone structure. But that is not the only space that we occupy. There is also our personal space. We have the experience of 'our' space being invaded when we feel that another person is standing too close. They are in our territory. How do we determine how close 'too close' is? That is less easily defined because it varies from person to person and can vary from time to time. Our awareness of another intruding into our space or our intruding into another's may be conscious or it may be subconscious. We may object to the person standing too close to us in line or we may feel vaguely irritable when chairs are placed very close to each other in a crowded meeting.

If we go into a library where there are just a few people, we will probably see several tables with just one person sitting at them. Chances are, if we look around and don't see anyone that we know, we too will pick an empty table. Or if we are sitting at a table and someone comes in and sits right next to us, when there are many other empty seats, we may feel annoyed, or at least wonder why. If the person is attractive to us and is someone we would like to know, then we will be pleased to share our space. Whatever our reaction is, it relates to our awareness or a feeling that we extend beyond our physical skin.

The air that we exhale mixes with the air that someone else inhales and so our air space mixes. The air that is outside of us one second is inside us the next second; what is outer becomes inner. We do not live encapsulated within our physical bodies. We can have the same experience with warmth. An uncomfortably cool room can become warm by people occupying it, or an already warm room can become too hot when occupied by several people. When a person is suffering from hypothermia after prolonged exposure to cold, the quickest treatment is to place him between two warm people. Both warmth and air are shared, and both are vital to our survival.

The way that surrounding space is arranged also affects us. From an awareness of this, concepts in architecture, landscaping, and decorating have developed. Our experience is different at the top of the mountain, than at the bottom, different in a cave or out at sea. We have an inner feeling that is not defined by measuring in inches. As parents we need to be aware that there is a reality to space and that it matters what space we create and provide for our child. We need to develop the artistic quality within us that helps us to be aware of the subtle, non-visible influences in our lives. For parenting we need to call on these artistic qualities in ourselves. We need to develop an awareness of space, our space, and others' space.

When we share the space of others who are happy, enjoying what they are doing and whom they are doing it with, we feel quite different from when we share space where there is conflict, anger, and disharmony. Worst of all is being in cold space, a place where there is a controlled absence of feelings. Then we shall probably feel inwardly cold, no matter how warm the room is. It is out of this coldness that hostility and cruelty can emerge.

The quality of the space surrounding a child has a strong effect on her; the infant and the toddler are especially vulnerable. Their senses are not so differentiated, they live in a totality, and absorb like a sponge what is around them. For them, what is outer becomes inner to a much stronger degree than it does for an adult. Remembering that we can feel the difference and how each different experience affects us, we can discover through our own observation what it will mean to the child. Through developing an awareness of the quality of space, we can then learn to create a harmonious nourishing environment.

An infant or toddler needs to be able to have a safe space that her parents create and share with her. In these first years she is still very dependent and needs to be a part of them, needs the protection that they can provide. By creating a space of peace for our child from infancy on, we are giving her a valuable gift, both physically and emotionally. The child has a lot of physical developing and growing to do and what happens in her environment affects how she grows and affects her health.

The way the body develops and grows is modified by what impinges upon it. Outer effects are fairly obvious, they are observable. The inner effects are less visible, but none the less observable. We are affected physically by our emotions. We can experience how our heart beat changes when we are really frightened, how our stomach 'knots' when we are the victim of someone's anger. We are familiar with the physical change that is apparent when we blush or turn pale. We can see the muscle tension that is associated with fear. When these changes are internal we can't observe their effects in the same way. It does seem reasonable to assume, however, that when organs have these experiences, there will also be some permanent effect.

Everyone's life is associated with some trauma and chaos and that is unavoidable. But if the environment is consistently destructive, then lasting effects will be inevitable. The important thing to know is that the environment matters. Feeling guilty when things go wrong does not help anyone. Being a caring person does help nourish those who are around us.

We know the pleasant experience of being in a warm caring environment. That is what we would like our apprentice to experience. A child who is accepted, cared for, allowed to unfold her own gifts and make her own discoveries, helped to learn about the world while having adults with balanced qualities to imitate, has a real head start on coping with the world.

Through infancy and during the time the child is developing her abilities to crawl, walk, and talk, she depends on us to be aware of her needs and provide for them. We need to learn to read the subtle clues that can direct us in her care. They don't come from a 'how to' book, they come from her. Establishing and maintaining a nourishing environment is a primary task of parents of the young child. She absorbs all that is around her. Our space is her space. She will show us in many ways that she wants us to be aware of her; to care for her; to be conscious of her. She needs the protection of sharing her naturalness, clarity and warmth. The more natural and comfortable the parent feels in the space the more nourishing it will be for the baby. When the child has developed the skill of walking and can explore with ease, the parents will allow the child to explore other space, still keeping the child in their consciousness, but allowing her to explore and experience. As the child learns other skills and independent play we will then help toward the experience of creating her own space. By allowing it, neither forcing it nor preventing it, we make it possible for the child to develop out of her own nature.

The child needs the opportunity to learn for herself; so that she can learn to know the world and be able to do the things that living in the world requires. Learning is enhanced when we can learn in an environment where the skills already exist. When the environment is familiar, when the parent performs the skill with ease, and allows the child to join in the task, the child is learning in the common family space and this is the most natural and effective way to learn.

When the child has the opportunity to learn about the world and to learn the skills necessary to function self-dependently in the world, she will feel comfortable in the world and will be able to become a productive citizen.

The child will want to help with tasks around the house at a fairly early age. Of course it is faster to do it yourself and exclude the child; but at what cost? The child is eager to learn about the world, and this quality of enthusiasm is an asset to maintain. The child learns best when eagerly participating in warm, friendly space.

As she develops her own skills and talents, she will be starting to create her own space. Through imitating those around her she will make attempts at establishing some independence and some separate space. To do this successfully, she needs to know that the space she shares with us is there for her to return to. We need to support and encourage this exploration in personal space. We don't want her to feel stranded but rather to feel understood. There will be many adventures away from our space and back into it again. This is a healthy experience for the child. As adults we can create together a space of peace to meet each other in the most human way, but for the child we need to be the creator of the common space. We will first provide common personal space and later she will be able to create her own appropriate space.

Learning takes place first in shared space, then in separate space.

We shall not discourage or impede her attempts at learning. We shall patiently allow her many attempts to learn to do things, and not instantly do it for her or take it away with annoyance, but allow her the opportunity to explore, practice and learn. What we think of as play for the child is just as serious to her as her life's work will be at a later age. Through her play, she is developing the basis for functioning in the world. We shall remember that what we know how to do in the world we also had to learn.

When we allow the child to live in her own space, then we give her the opportunity for inner discovery. It is an important gift allowing her to learn to do things on her own, to develop her own capabilities and to develop a sense of competence. We don't want to force her into this at too early an age, neither do we want to take the experience away from her when she is ready to unfold it. If we are in tune with our child we will be able to know when it is time, based not on when we want her to do it, but when she is ready out of her own capacities.

If we smother the child with care and attention or we desert her and leave her on her own, we are not providing her with what she needs to become a functioning person in the world. Just as the seedling with too much or too little sun or water cannot grow in the best way; so the child also needs the right balance and intermix of care and attention, shared space and private space, for her optimum development.

First the child needs space that is created and protected by the parents. A space that is comfortable, with others. We do have to choose the part of the task that is safe and appropriate for the child to do, we need to show her the right way to do it, and then we need to step out of her space and allow her to do it. The child is a most generous fellow and delights in doing things for us and helping us. She, too, wants to be a part of the world and share in it. It is very tempting to put our hands in the child's space and take over the task when she struggles with it. But stop. Rather show her again: by watching you do the task she sees how it is done and can imitate it. Let her have the chance to build some talents in her own space. We want her to learn these skills that we have learned so that later she can give them back to the world, not to make us proud of her, nor to please us, but to allow her to learn what needs to be learned in our world. We can be pleased together and proud together as new skills are acquired. The child needs the opportunity to learn for herself; so that she can know the world and be able to do the things that living in the world requires. Through successful experiences we develop a sense of competence, a feeling that we can manage and function in the world.

Through our life's experiences we develop our own self image. The child's personality will be the sum total of all these experiences, plus her own individuality. It is with our personality that we meet the world, it becomes an important part of living. To approach the world with confidence and a feeling of self dependence is a valuable asset.

Physical aspects of space are important as well as the emotional aspects. Natural light and fresh air are natural elements for healthy living. As much as possible allow the child to enjoy natural light both outdoors and coming in through the windows. It is an unfortunate habit that has us close the curtains and then turn on the lights. Natural light is health-giving. Dress the child warmly enough so that the house does not have to be unpleasantly hot. Open the windows and doors in the morning so the fresh morning air can come in. Clean, fresh air is health-giving. The air in homes becomes stale if they are always closed up. The whole family will feel better if the new air of a new day circulates within the house.

Smoke-filled rooms, insect spray, and insect strips are all unnecessary poisons that have no place in the space of a child. There is no point in burdening them with unhealthy air and poisons. Rather allow them the opportunity to grow and develop in a healthy growing environment.

There are many things that are important in our personal space. When our astronauts went to the moon, they had to take their personal space needs with them to outer space. It is earth space that our earth bodies need to survive. Although the body can compensate for distortions and survive when the basic needs are not met, it is at a sacrifice. Children who have been under-nourished from birth may live, but they are unable to manifest their own abilities in the way a child can who has been properly nourished.

When we gain a feeling for personal space then we shall be considerate of the other person's space, both physically and emotionally. We shall provide a safe space, both physically and emotionally. A safe space for the child will nourish her so that she can live and grow with her wholeness. By having the experience of a warm, loving, protected safe space, she will have the opportunity to develop her capacities to the fullest and as she grows she will be able to stand upright in her own space and later build a space of peace with others.

8. The artificial world

As we look at the world, we are amazed by what our children need to learn. Once upon a time, and not so very long ago, all we needed to know to survive in the world were the local customs, local laws, and to learn a skill that was needed locally. We would probably go to the same church that our family attended, vote for the same party in elections, perhaps carry on the tasks of our parents, and in general by the time we reached adulthood, we would know our own personal world. But now we are asked to be citizens of the whole world, to make decisions that were previously made by professionals and to make choices that previously did not exist. It is no longer enough to provide our children with the right answers, they must be able to find the right questions. Life has become so complex and diversified that to understand it, we must learn to ask the right questions, find the right answers and then be able to make reasoned choices. The choices that we make, the things we say 'yes' to and the things we say 'no' to help create our individual path through life.

The skills needed for making choices are many, starting with the ability to sort out what the choices are. We have to have some understanding of the consequences and decide which we with our own unique individuality can best live with. Life is not problem-free, ever. We just decide which problems we prefer to live with. When we look at the world and our choices, we need to know if we are being realistic, if we are putting the facts together as they really exist. Is the information that we have true, does it correspond to the facts?

Finding truth and reality has also become more difficult as the world has become more complex. There was a time when if you were given a planter with a plant in it you knew you would have to care for it. You would put it near a light source, water it regularly, neither too much nor too little, and feed it occasionally. You would have to get to know the plant; 'read' its signals to you, to take care of it.

Today it is quite possible that the plant you get will not need you or your care. It may be plastic. It will survive, unchanged, without any help from you or anyone else. It will not wilt, die, or grow. The way it is, is the way it will always be. It doesn't matter if it is put in the sun, or the shade, the environment will not impinge on the plant or interact with it; it will not produce the oxygen that a living plant will, and it will not moderate the humidity; the interaction of plant and man will not occur. Through the wisdom of nature, man inhales oxygen and exhales carbon dioxide, the plant absorbs the carbon dioxide and transforms it into oxygen. With plastic plants this does not occur. To external observation both plants may appear the same. The plastic plant may be so cleverly made that there are brown tips on some of the leaves to make it look 'real'. What is 'real' and what is 'not real'? If it looks real from the outside, does that make it real? How does a natural growing plant differ from a plastic one? How does a mannequin differ from a living person? Unreal imitations can be so cleverly done that they are hard to distinguish by a quick glance. If we only look at the external, visible aspects of anything we may be deceived. If we observe carefully with an attempt at understanding the nature and dynamics inherent in the object, deception is no longer possible.

Part of the reality of our world is that an ever-growing portion of it is plastic. How has it changed our view of reality? Is plastic real? Is a plastic glass, a glass? Is a plastic flower, a flower? Does it smell, grow, die? Is wood-grained printed plastic panelling wood panelling? When we look at a table can we tell if it is plastic or wood? Have you had the conversation, 'Is it all right to put the drink on the table?' and been told, 'Yes, it doesn't matter, it is plastic.'?

What is being said when we say it doesn't matter? It doesn't matter what happens to the table? No, we are saying, it won't hurt the table, it doesn't matter what you do, you don't need to care for it. The ads say, 'Care-free plastic, stain resistant, rustproof, unbreakable'. What does that mean? What can we learn from plastics? We learn how easily we are deceived by outer appearances, by outer clues. We learn that we have little or no effect on them. We learn that natural laws do not affect them. We learn that we do not matter, our caring is not needed.

When what you do does not matter, what happens? You don't need to care for things. You are not acknowledged by the world around you. Your presence is not counted. This tells us that man is not important, we don't matter. We don't need to do anything to care for them. We may as well not be there.

Plastic is there and it doesn't change. It does not tell us anything about the laws of nature and the interactions in the world. Nature transforms natural products and we can learn nature's secrets by observing. If we put garbage in the ground in a short time it is no longer visible and becomes a part of the earth. If we have a compost pile and combine garbage, manure, soil, straw, we are rewarded with sweet-smelling fertile soil. One of nature's mysteries.

We cannot learn about the laws of nature from plastics. They do not share the secret wisdom of nature, they tell us we don't matter. They leave man as unimportant. Plastic is there and it doesn't change, it resists the changes inherent in nature. It dulls our capacity for observation because there are no subtle changes. When we make the choice to live with plastics and synthetics, are we aware of the consequences?

Baby drops his plastic bottle on the floor, it won't break, so it does not matter. He drops his plastic glass on the floor, it won't break, it doesn't matter. What he does, doesn't matter. He doesn't need to be careful. But the truth is that people need to matter and we also need to develop the feeling of caring for things. It is through caring that we can learn about things and develop an interest in them. The world needs caring people.

If we live only with things that make us say, it doesn't matter; in fact it won't matter. Plastic is separate and stays separate. It does not interact with other substances. Spill latex-based paint on a nylon rug and what happens? Nothing — it doesn't matter. Just wipe up the paint. The paint does not affect the rug. There is no exchange of colour or substance. The paint yields nothing to the rug, the rug yields nothing to the paint. Great, you think. But at what cost? Can it be all good, with no problems?

No, it can't. We have made a choice. We have brought into our lives something that makes us not matter. Our children live with us in an environment where things don't matter and people don't matter. We learn not to care for things, and then we have created a non-caring environment for the people who live there. We have created an environment of isolation — one thing does not affect another, and soon that affects people. What do we feel when we say, we don't care, it doesn't matter? The feeling that comes with that is separation, disinterest, apathy, eventually contempt. Our feelings are real. They live with us and go with us every day. They go everywhere we go. It is not possible to feel contempt for something you have cared for and have become interested in. You can feel frustration, anger, annoyance, but not contempt.

A child absorbs the emotional environment that he lives in. Everything affects him. There is nothing that happens that does not matter, that does not affect him.

Perhaps we then decide that we want our child to learn how to take care of things; to feel that he matters. He throws the plastic cup on the floor. We say, 'no', but if it is empty and cannot break, is it a reasonable 'no'? We say 'no', but it is hard to make it matter. If it won't break and does not need to be cared for, why shouldn't he throw it? Now where are we? We can't tell him, 'no', it will break. That isn't true. We can say it isn't nice, but that is a pretty empty arbitrary judgment based on no visible reality. By having the safe, convenient plastic bottle we have put the child and ourselves in a position of living the reality that what he does and what we do, in this case at least, does not matter. There is no way that we can pretend that dropping it or throwing it does matter. Inevitably, he will eventually learn not to care for things, which leads to contempt.

After the Second World War when plastics first appeared in the stores, the natural question was, 'Is it real or is it plastic?' Another thought was that it looked too perfect to be real. At that time there was a consciousness that there was a difference between a natural product and a machine-made artificial one. Being perfect and identical were not viewed as something to strive for. When most things were made of natural materials by people using machines, the sameness of plastic items was more observable. As we have more and more plastics, the basis for discrimination is lost, the opportunity for observation is gone.

But we are still faced with the need to make a choice. Plastic things are cheaper and don't need to be cared for. Some people will take that as the most important consideration and opt for plastic. Others have a feeling for man-made things of natural fabrics and materials, a feeling that what is made by man for man is somehow special. That special feeling is there each time the item is seen or used. This is not something that is called home-made because it is poorly done. It is an item made with care by an experienced craftsman who has developed this human talent into a skill, or made with care by a loving one.

The comparatively low cost of plastics is a dilemma. That seems like a strange thing to worry about in our inflationary times. To find anything that is cheap seems like a relief, but what problems does that lead to? It leads to another 'it doesn't matter', because we can easily buy another one. Not only do we not matter now, but neither does the object. Everything is replaceable. We will be able to find an exact duplicate — or a million machine-made copies if we choose.

The process continues: People in the world don't matter. It takes very few people to make plastic items; so the profits are high. Economists tell us that it is labour-intensive products that are expensive. That could ultimately lead to machines doing the work and men walking around, unemployed, unneeded and in despair. Do we know what we are doing to ourselves, and is it what we want?

We think that it is our money that buys the things and totally forget about all the people that are involved in the process. How much more it means to a child if we tell him about the man who planted and cared for the trees, the sun and rain that helped them grow, the logger who cut them down, the lumberman who sorted, dried, and milled the wood, the craftsman who made the article, the storeman who bought it from the craftsman, and the truck driver who delivered it to the store. He then knows about all the people who worked together so that he could have the toy. Then the world becomes real, with real people doing real deeds.

When the world we live in reveals the laws of nature to us, we can develop our powers of observation and learn to understand causes. We have a chance to connect apparently separate phenomena. The plant is not watered and it will droop, and if we don't see the cause and still don't water it, it dies. Our observation matters and we matter.

We learn to ask questions, to observe causes and see that we do have choices. We care for the plant, water it and it stays with us. We can make choices and our choices affect the world.

By living with observing, caring parents, children learn to observe and care, they learn to ask questions, identify causes, find answers, and to make choices based on reason.

9. Truth and reality

We choose our path as we go through life and create a path for our children. When our path is clearly defined, consistent, and thoughtfully chosen, our children will benefit. The world they live in is clearer for them, and without distortions. If we are to understand the world we have to develop abilities for uncluttered looking and quiet listening.

Often our looking takes on a hurried superficial glimpse: how easy it is to miss the significant realities if we do not see past the external appearances. It is through conscious observation that we can develop an understanding of the world and what is in it.

When we combine salt and water in appropriate ratios, we have a new substance with new properties, saline solution. If we evaporate the water, we can again recognize the salt. Salt, a visible crystalline substance becomes invisible when it is dissolved in water, and can become visible again through evaporation of the water.

Water that was visible becomes invisible as it is heated and evaporates. A dynamic interaction occurs that is measurable and predictable. It is dependable, yet changeable. It combines and it separates. Through observation we can learn about the laws of nature.

If we make water cold enough it will freeze, become hard and solid and lose its ability to flow. If we heat it sufficiently it will disperse in a gaseous state. It is affected by its environment. It goes from a hardened separate form, through a flowing intermingling, to invisibility by dispersion.

Although water is usually taken for granted and not the object of observation, it is a remarkable substance, with hidden mysteries to be discovered. It assumes a form when it is frozen, it is formless at warmer temperatures, and evaporates at still higher temperatures. When the sun shines on the little drops at a certain angle, we see the magnificent colours of the rainbow. Water in a flowing stream or bubbling spring is vibrantly alive, reflecting the light as it dances down its path. Water in a stagnant pool is dull and cloudy. How much there is to learn about nature by really observing water.

Water is not only a separate, directly visible element. Water and its effects can be observed in plants, animals and man. Life depends on water. By observing a waterless desert that is barren of plant and animal life we are led to think of the importance of water for living things, perhaps the bearer of a life substance. Man can survive for a much longer time without food than he can without water. Through what we learn by observing water, we can better understand the world of nature and of man.

When we say she is 'cold as ice', or to be careful you will get in 'hot water', we are using our awareness of the natural world to understand human situations. By observing the natural world around us and developing an understanding of it we can develop our capacities for seeing the reality in the world.

Finding reality in the world is a significant yet difficult thing to do. We have looked at the artificial man-created world and discovered that educating our sense perceptions is another task in life. Can we distinguish between plastic leather and leather, synthetic wool and wool, wood-printed plastic and wood? Without accurate perceptions, knowing what we are seeing, we are missing the first step in understanding. We first need a clear perception to combine with the appropriate descriptive or explanatory concept. We need to link true perceptions and true concepts to find reality. We need to complete the unfinished portion of what we see.

There was a time when truth was taken for granted. It was seen as an honourable quality and expected of those that were respected in the world. Words were used with more care, and knowingly distorting the truth was not accepted. Somewhere along the way the rationalization that 'it is only a white lie', and the 'end justifies the means', crept into our thinking and put us to sleep. What is a white lie? It is an untruth. If it is not true, it is not true. Truth does not come in increments, it is whole. We have become clever with thoughts and words and in so doing we have lost the sense for truth. To have a sense for truth and to recognize an untruth requires living with the truth. Children when they are young do this quite naturally. But if we ask them to be clever, and they see us being clever, they will lose their natural truthfulness.

To avoid an unpleasant situation, an untruth may be used. When we don't have the courage to live with reality or when we want to create our own reality, we may lie. Perhaps we don't want to say 'no' to the salesman at the door or on the telephone, so we tell the child to tell the caller we are not home. Remembering that the child internalizes his environment, what are we teaching? How can he learn to be truthful when his world is not truthful and we ask him to be a part of that world? To develop a sense for truth and recognize untruth requires living with the truth. Once you are off on the path of the artful dodger or deceiver, you lose the natural ability. You may even lose that inner feeling that makes you uneasy when you are not telling the truth.

It is easy to be led into an untruth with the excuse that you do not want to hurt the other person's feelings. A point to remember is that you don't have to say anything. You can keep your opinion to yourself. If the other person really needs to know, then you are really hurting them more by speaking an untruth. Truth may be painful, but it is never harmful if it is thoughtfully and kindly given. Remember the thoughtful and kindly part.

Somewhere along the way in our social evolution we acquired the misperception that cleverness was a desirable trait to acquire. When we say, 'isn't that clever!' it has a certain approval. We may enjoy knowing clever people and want to own clever things. What is cleverness?

The magician shows us, it is his stock in trade. The magician is in the world to show us that we can be tricked into non-reality through cleverness. As we watch a magician, we know we are being deceived. He is showing us that he is so clever that our senses can be tricked into thinking something untrue is true. It is a game between us and the magician and we both enjoy it. Remember the things that the magician teaches us. Remember that what we think is real, may not be. We may be dreaming our way through a life that is a hoax. Keep asking. Is it true, is it real, is it right? When we see that something is clever, or easy, or tricky, ask what the deception is, and what problems go with not knowing what is true.

The magician is honest with us. He tells us he plans to trick us. He doesn't deceive us into thinking that he is showing us truth and reality. In fact he lets us know that it is not real. He tells us he is going to be clever and he is going to make us think something is true that is not. How do we identify the magicians of the world who are not so honest with us? How do we develop the ability to discriminate reality and non-reality in the world? Can we be alert to the world magicians without going through life being suspicious? Can we refine our own perceptions of the world and learn to discriminate and evaluate?

It is through our feelings that we can sense truth and untruth, reality and non-reality. We can develop a feeling for truth and reality and when we combine it with our reason, we learn to understand what is happening in the world. Feelings must be educated and developed just as thinking is. It is only when our feelings are acknowledged and allowed that they be-

110

come a functioning part of our personality. It is with our feelings that we interact with the world, we feel connected with each other.

We may describe a person as warm-hearted, lively, or compassionate, or as a free soul. Then we are talking about the person who trusts and allows his feelings to tell him about the world. When we speak of someone as being up-tight, we think of someone who is uncomfortable with his feelings.

If we are going to help our children grow up to be the whole human beings that they can be, then we will allow them their feelings. That does not mean that we will ask the small child to become conscious of his feelings. It means that we become aware of the value of having feelings and we respect the feelings of others. It is when our feelings are allowed that we can learn to recognize and identify them. We ask each other all the time, 'How do you feel?' or 'How are you?' Unfortunately, that is not usually a 'real' question and we are expected to say, 'Just fine'. That seems to be acknowledging the existence of feelings without the willingness to allow real feelings.

It is important to recognize the value of feelings, and to know how we can use them. Part of the adult maturing process is to get in touch with our own feelings, learn from them, but not be manipulated by them. We need to balance our feelings and our reason. If they can be made conscious, then we can discover what battle is being waged within ourselves: the struggle between our ideas, our reason and our desires. If a child has the opportunity to live with people who recognize their own feelings and do not overwhelm

111

others with them, then the child has a head start on finding reality in the world

Allowing our feelings, identifying them and educating them takes some sorting out that can be a bit puzzling. It requires discriminating among feelings, desires and emotions. Frequently these words are used interchangeably, but there are differences and we shall try to clarify those differences.

Feelings are universal and varied. There is joy, sorrow, fear, wonder, reverence, peace, boredom, enthusiasm, and so on. There are body postures that typically go with each of these feelings. When we see someone walking down the street, with head down, shoulders hunched, and a smile on their face, we become concerned about the incongruity. We think that there is something wrong with the person. Feelings are inner experiences, but we can learn to recognize them in others as well as in ourselves. There are common identifiable feelings in the world.

Feelings do become individualized. Most people feel a warmth and happiness at parties and weddings, excitement at sports events, and reverence in a beautiful church. But the usual feelings are not inevitable and will be affected by our own desires. If we didn't want the people to get married, we might be sad instead of happy.

We associate 'I want' with desires. It is a self centred experience. Please remember, not good or bad, but different. We do not learn about reality from desires, we learn about ourselves and what pleases us. We find what we like and how we want the world to be, what makes us happy or unhappy.

As if that were not complicated enough, we also have emotions and they are a bit different. Being an emotional person is not the same as being a feeling person. Feelings are inwardly experienced and contained. Emotions overflow, they are more visible reactions, they are separate and belong to the person who is having them. Feelings are shared, they are common realities that we can learn to recognize. We may feel anger at injustice: if we rage about it, the feeling of anger has become emotional rage; then the tendency is to react out of the emotion. By recognizing our feeling of anger, not repressing it, we can acknowledge it and learn from it. And when we develop that self control we are strengthening our individual self.

We want our apprentice to have experiences that will allow for a variety of feelings. We especially want the child to be able to experience wonder and reverance and caring. When he sees us feeling sorrow at others' misfortune, joy at the sunrise, wonder at the beauty of springtime and reverence for all living things then his feelings are being educated in reality.

For those who are concerned about man's inhumanity to man, about the faceless masses, about people who don't want to get involved, we need to take a clear look at what we are doing in our own lives daily that is encouraging the very thing we don't want to bring into the world. How can we get back to truth, reality and reasoned choices? We can help our children by providing them with real-life experiences, with natural consequences and an environment where natural laws can be observed, where human dignity and human needs are respected. If they have

113

lived with truth and reality, they will have the chance to recognize it in the world and to distinguish it from untruth and non-reality. We will then have given them a valuable treasure. They will then learn to ask, 'Is it true? Is it real? Is it right?' Through our knowing what is true and what is real we can find our own real path through the world and then we are more able to create a path for our children. We will be providing them with the basis of good mental health. When we have clear perceptions, active thinking and feeling, and the ability to work in the world, we can recognize truth, and live in reality. Then we live as mature stable adults who can handle what comes to us on our path through life.

10. The handicapped child

If you have a child with a handicap you are well aware that you have to make some adjustments in your parenting role; your child will need some special care. The adjustments and differences, however, are less than the similarities.

The child is still a unique individual, no matter what the handicap. She has feelings that are her own and are important. She too will develop best if given loving care, warmth, and is allowed to be herself. However, our world may be more complex and perplexing to her and difficult for her to sort out, know, and understand. It is quite likely that her sense perceptions are different from ours. She might be more sensitive to noise, light, or other disturbances around her or it is possible that some of her senses are more acute and some more dulled than usual. You will have to develop more finely attuned abilities of observation, because a handicap is usually associated with an inability to sort out and express needs in as clear a way. Be aware of her reactions so that you know what is stressful for her. Her sense of touch may be more acute. Her ability to maintain body warmth may be diminished and she may require extra clothing.

Chances are that you will know your child better and in a more meaningful way than the experts you will want to consult to provide the extra help your child will need. The professionals will know more about the condition and treatment but you will know more about your individual child. You will need more ability than the usual parent to be able to sort out what is fact from what is fiction and prejudice. Once you have separated fact from theory it will be up to you to decide what is the human thing to do with the facts. You will have to be able to put yourself in the role of the child and ask, 'If this were me, what would I want done?' By putting away any feelings of sympathy, or feeling sorry for her, and working out of compassion, you will give the gift to your child, whatever the handicap, of having the opportunity to grow in whatever way she can: to allow her to develop her potential. We need to discover what is right for the child as she is and not lament over what she is not. Remember: not, 'better or worse than,' but 'unique and different'. That is just as true of handicapped people as it is of anyone else.

Some children have minor handicaps and some children's handicaps are more global. You will want all the expertise you can gain, you will want to call on professionals, and you will benefit from getting to know other families with handicapped children. But when all is said and done, it will be your decision what kind of life your child will have.

There are a variety of services available to handicapped children and their families and it is important to know of the resources available to you. In most countries free education is a right for all handicapped children. Thanks to the dedicated work and persistence of parents of handicapped children and the professionals who have worked with them, the opportunities available to them have increased. Get to know the schools in your area, as well as what is being provided elsewhere. You too can work to improve the quality of the services available, just as before you parents of handicapped children worked to establish them. It is important to remember that, whatever the handicap, she too needs to be able to learn about and function in the world to the degree that she is able.

Often having a child with a handicap is the parent's first introduction into the world of the handicapped. Initially it is a shock, and it takes some real sorting out of human values, spiritual values, and social values. More often than not parents of handicapped children, once they have gone through the first emotional reactions and sorted out the realities, find their experience in the world of the handicapped to be one of the most meaningful of their lives. Not that the child is lucky to be handicapped, but that parents quickly learn that there is much more to a child than the external physical appearance.

With the handicapped child, developmental milestones are measured in smaller increments. Her timetable may be different, but her developmental sequences will be the same. It will be important to separate her developmental age from her chronological age. Old prejudices die hard, but it is important to recognize a thirty-year-old handicapped person with the dignity of an adult in an adult world and not treat her as an eternal child. That she is not.

Some handicapped children are not able to give

their parents the clues that healthy children are able to give. They may not cry when they are cold or hungry and you will have to be more aware and observant in their care.

If your child is mentally retarded she will still learn by imitation, but she will probably need to have more repetition and a clearer structure. She too will need a path that is familiar, consistent, reliable, and a family that is warm and loving, because she will understand that very well. She also is an apprentice to the world and will need you to help her gain all the skills that she will need for living in the world. She will be able to learn when she has a good teacher. She will always learn best by being shown what to do, a step at a time; by imitating what she observes. One young lady put it so well when she told me, 'I'm not dumb you know, just slow.'

If her sense perceptions are affected then we need to understand how this affects her development and find ways to help her learn to bypass the missing perception.

For the blind child, we help her use her hands to identify the world. Most of us learn to know about the world through looking at it. We recognize familiar objects and learn their names. It is important to understand what it is like to not see the world or to see the world distorted. Our balance, in part, is developed from visual clues. The child that cannot see will inevitably feel more separated. However, she can learn from verbal clues that she is not alone. Parents can talk to her more often than usual when they are in the same room, or they can hum or sing.

When you hold a blind child, put her hand on your face, hair, neck; blow on her hand, so that her hands will help her bring parts of the outer world to her. Allow her to sense the world through her hands. When she progresses to the crawling stage she will usually be reassured if at first she is in a playpen and can identify her boundaries in all directions. Exploring will be a safer experience for her if she can establish that she can return to something familiar.

A suggestion that you may want to try when she is learning to walk is tying a ribbon around her waist and attaching it securely to something about five feet away. Then with one hand she can hold onto her ribbon and feel secure in her further explorations. You will want to hold her hand when she walks, as you would for any child, and describe verbally what she is doing: stepping up, stepping down, stopping, opening the door, or whatever it is.

The first words that children learn are nouns, names of things and people. It is very difficult to have a meaningful vocabulary if you don't know what the word describes. To help her when she is learning to talk, let her hold the object that you are naming, so that she can associate the word with the object. When you say 'bye', move her hand in a waving motion, realizing that she cannot see your gestures.

Familiar smells will be an important part of the environment for a blind child. You might want to put a dish of cloves in one room, a dish of cinnamon in another room; so that she can recognize different places through her sense of smell.

When she seems fearful it may help to bring her

119

hands together for her, holding them in yours. By touching her one hand with the other she can have a feeling of being contained.

Talk to her from a distance as you approach her and keep talking as you come closer so that she can learn to discriminate distance through sound. When you get next to her, touch her as you speak.

Let her know that she is living with a family that loves and accepts her and she will smile.

For the deaf child we are aware of how separate and isolated she feels because she cannot communicate through listening and we shall work at communicating with her in other ways. By increasing our touching and eye contact we shall reassure her that she is part of our world and we are part of hers. In our culture speech is our primary method of communication and we forget how much we can relate to each other through gestures, body posture, and visual clues. It will be important to establish these other methods of communication. Communication is a primary concern even though it cannot be verbal communication. Look for agencies that provide specialized services and start a course in total communication so that as your child grows you can help her learn about the world. She will need the opportunity to learn alternative methods of communication so that she can get to know about the world and the people in it, and so that she can tell others what is meaningful to her.

If the child has a chronic illness, learn as much as you can about it and then build as normal a life as possible within the constraints of the illness. You will need to avoid the tendency of being over-protective and allow the child the opportunity to develop at whatever rate is possible for her. Work to know what her limitations are and what you can do to help overcome them. It is important to get to know the child as she is, the real her, and not think of her as a 'defective' model of what your fantasy is that she 'should' be. Avoid any preconceived ideas of what her eventual limitations will be, but accept the current realities of her handicap.

One of the primary things you can give your child is the feeling that you accept her totally as she is, just as you want others to accept you as you are.

She is a total person, a unique individuality with feelings and thoughts. Even if she can't express them, she still has them. The attitude of the people around her will affect her strongly. Somewhere we came up with the misconception that the only things inside a person are what we can pull out. We test to measure knowledge. The trouble is we might not know enough to ask all the right questions.

There is unmistakable evidence that receptive language is not limited by expressive language. The profoundly disabled child needs to be talked to, read to, and included in family-style living. We cannot risk setting limitations on what we think the child is taking in because we can be completely wrong. Our moods, our gestures, and our deeds will all be important. We can think of the child as a musician with a damaged instrument. No matter how much a great violinist knows about playing a violin, if the violin is damaged, distorted sounds will be heard. The violinist will not be able to share with us all of his talents, because the damaged instrument limits him. In the same way, we cannot judge the abilities of the handicapped child by what she communicates to us, because her physical instrument is damaged. It is her body, not her uniqueness or her feelings, that is handicapped.

For the handicapped child it is even more essential to allow her to live with a rhythmic day that is consistent, in an environment of optimism. She, too, needs to be allowed to develop all that she is capable of. We need only read the biography of Helen Keller to develop an awe of the heroic accomplishments of handicapped people. To know their indomitable courage and endurance can be an important lesson for us. To share their feeling of satisfaction at the smallest accomplishment can make us realize how much we take for granted in life.

If you are not a parent of a handicapped child, but a neighbour or friend of one, then help your child to understand that the handicap is only a small part of the child, and much more importantly she is a fellow human being, with feelings, and desires and needs for friends and activities. She needs to be welcomed into the world, too, and allowed to live in dignity out of her own humanness.

We all have things that we do well and things that we struggle with, but for some what we struggle with is not as visible. What matters is that we do whatever we can in the best way we can. We work with ourselves as we are and try to become what is possible, despite our handicap, large or small.

11. Independence versus freedom

A recurring theme throughout history has been man's search for freedom. Courageous people have chosen to endure hardship and danger in the hope of finding a place to live in freedom; freedom from oppression, freedom to worship, to live in dignity, to seek their own path. Throughout history people have left familiar lands and their families in search of a place where they could fulfil their dreams, dreams of freedom and justice. Wars have been fought as whole countries have struggled to be free.

What is this search for freedom, what does it mean to be free? When we think of freedom we think of an inner experience, an opportunity to choose for ourselves without compulsion; a chance to allow and to explore our own thoughts, our own feelings, our own dreams. When we make choices without the restriction of following the long list of 'shoulds' in the world or doing what we feel compelled to do by our own needs and desires we experience freedom. Being free means we are in touch with our feelings, but we do not react out of them. We listen to and accept and we think about how we feel. Our actions do not occur uncontrolled or independent of our own combined thinking and feeling. We also think about others, about man-made laws and rules, expectations, and then we do what we feel is right, what is right out of our own ethical moral philosophy. Freedom relates to our making a responsible choice about our own life style and allowing others to choose theirs.

It soon becomes clear that responsibility is the companion of freedom. If we are going to choose our own path through life, then we take full responsibility for our actions and do not excuse or justify what we do. We don't expect to be perfect, but we do expect to try our utmost to do what is right and good. We make responsible inner decisions, neither following our desires and drives nor other people's expectations of us. When we associate responsibility with freedom, then we can differentiate licence from freedom. Freedom does not mean to do anything we please; it means to stand in balance in our own space and choose what we feel is right. This is what we want our apprentice to learn to do for himself as an adult. Freedom cannot be given to us, it is an inner experience, but it can be allowed.

How does freedom differ from independence? It is possible to discount the difference and say it is only a question of semantics. Then what are we saying? We are avoiding looking at the difference or pretending that it is the word, not the situation that we are trying to understand; so that is no real answer. Somehow the inner yearning for freedom drifted to the thought of independence. How do they differ? When we describe someone as being independent we usually think of someone who takes care of himself, feels he does not need others, perhaps he does not consider others, does things his own way and takes care of number one. He may be described as proud or a self-made man. To be independent is to be separate from, to be on one's own. We are individuals and we are separate. We have our own space, our own needs, and our own goals. As our apprentice grows into adolescence he develops more of his separate identity; so he has new needs. In his childhood he learned through imitation, in his early school years he searched for the authorities in the world, 'my dad said', 'my teacher said': he looks up to heroes and he needs heroes.

In adolescence we find our apprentice seeking for true information, reason, good judgment. He no longer just accepts what is around him, or believes what anyone says, he wants to test things out for himself. Geometry and mathematics are good examples of a reality that he can come to through his own understanding. The laws of mathematics and measurements are true and can be worked out for himself. If he has learned how to observe, he can discover for himself the true laws of nature. He wants to understand the world out of his own inner qualities and separateness. He needs a basis for his decisions and choices. The world he sees may be a painful experience for him. If he had the opportunity to experience joy and wonder and reverence in his childhood and he has learned skills for caring for himself and others, he will have the inner qualities necessary to meet the demands of growing into a less than perfect adult world. If he has learned what is true, learned to observe and connect causes, he has a way of making his own decisions.

He will begin to experience times when he feels inwardly free to make independent judgments in the world and have a sense of what it means to be really human. When decisions are made and opinions are held without a real understanding of the situation, prejudices follow. Adolescents have the task of getting to know themselves as individuals seeking a place in the world. We have the task of preparing them for this and allowing it.

As our apprentice matures, becomes more of an individual, using his own abilities to make independent judgments, he experiences this separateness. My thoughts and feelings and ways of doing things may not be yours. I am uniquely me and you are uniquely you. But can we be independent?

Even though we may think of ourselves as independent, in fact we are really dependent on each other and the world. Farmers, truckers, builders, plumbers, electricians, teachers, doctors, dentists, ministers, policemen, firemen, secretaries, artists, musicians — the list goes on and on — all play an important part in our lives. We may make our own clothes, but do we grow the cotton, care for the sheep, spin, weave and dye the cloth we use? We need each other. We depend on each other.

We see that each person takes on a task in life and then shares the fruits of his labour. One person develops the skill of car maintenance, another grows vegetables, another raises cattle, someone mines ore, someone works in the steel mills, someone makes the car parts. In our complicated society one person cannot accomplish all the complex tasks for himself.

It could be argued that we don't need to learn to do these things, because we have money and can buy what we want and there are machines to do all the work, automatically, and there are computers to replace our memory. But computers do not make new discoveries, they can only retrieve or rearrange past information that man has put into them and retrieve it in the way he has told them to. Computers sort and recall. They are not creative and cannot discover. They do not contribute to the evolutionary process.

Do not be deceived into thinking that if you pay money for the things you use that you are providing for yourself. Without the deeds of our fellow man and our ancestors most of us would have a difficult time surviving in the world. It is important to remember that money is a means of exchange, it may represent someone's deeds, but it is not a deed.

Total independence is really not an option; so how dependent do we want to be on others? It is a matter of degree, of balance, again. The more basic skills we have learned, the more self-dependent we can become; not independent, but self-dependent. Generally an exchange of money goes with an exchange of skills. The fewer skills that we have the more money we need to have things done for us. The more skills that we have the more self-reliant we can be and the less vulnerable we are to the economic system. The less we provide for ourselves, the more money we need and the more estranged we become from the world we live in.

We expect the child to be dependent on his family while he is learning skills for living in the world. We take responsibility for him and provide for him while he learns about the world and about himself. We give him the opportunity to get to know himself and find his relationship in the world. This extra time for learning is unique to man. In the animal world the young very quickly learn how to care for themselves in the world.

As the child's sense of responsibility develops we allow opportunities for him to experience the meaning of caring for himself. We guide and provide opportunities for him to work toward self-dependence with responsibility. By living with caring people he learns to be a caring person; to care for himself, others, and the world. By living with morality, he learns what morality is.

When we are self-dependent we can choose what we do for ourselves, what we do for others and what we ask others to do for us. Then we are able to share in life with others. We do not exclude or ignore the other fellow, nor do we use or manipulate him. It will be clear to us that everyone matters and we have learned to be carers, producers, consumers, and givers.

Everything that we give to a machine to do, we take away from the activity of a man. The humanness is removed. Somewhere the untrue idea was promoted that inactivity and the easy way were the ideal state for man: nothing to do, all of your needs met and you just sit around. To be part of the idle rich somehow was promoted as the good life. That is so far from true it is hard to understand how it got such a firm hold on thinking. Rather it is activity that is synonymous with being human. Creativity is a reward of being human. Feeling responsible and self-dependent allows us to discover our humanness. We have heard the lament of recently retired people who are bored, and depressed by their feeling of uselessness. These same people who were looking forward to being idle as their reward for having spent their lives working. Overwork, all work and no play, might make one think one would prefer idleness, but what is really needed is the right balance between work and play. Time to work, time to play, and time to rest.

It is when we have mastered life's basic skills, that we can become self-dependent. Being self-dependent means depending on ourselves. It does not mean thinking that we don't need others.

We want our apprentice to develop self-dependence. We want him to develop skills in building, farming, cooking, cleaning, sewing, to learn how to provide for basic food, clothing, and shelter. We want him to learn how to care for things. By developing these skills, he is given an opportunity to know and understand the world that he lives in. Then he will not feel isolated and estranged. He will be able to care for himself and to help others.

The more skills for living that we help our children acquire, the better equipped they will be to understand the world. When we know how to grow our own foods, and cook or bake, then we develop an understanding and appreciation for the foods that we eat and for the people who provide them for us. When we know how to sew, knit, weave, crochet, wash, and iron our clothes, then we know and understand about our clothing, how it has been made and how to care for it. If we have learned about plumbing and electricity, if we can repair the equipment that we have, if we understand how our automobile works, we will be less a stranger in the world that we live in. Then we will be able to experience it as a friendly place to be in, and we can become self-dependent. We will be able to depend upon ourselves, to provide for and care for ourselves. We can live in the world with a feeling of confidence, not separated from the world but as a part of it and then we will be able to function in it.

As we learn to appreciate our fellow man in the world, we will strive for self-dependence, not independence. We need to care for others and to be cared for. We are nourished by the warm feelings that come with caring and being cared for, we need to unfold our humanness. That is not possible when we are alone, separate and independent, thinking only of ourselves. When we are independent and self-concerned we are estranged from others, pleasing ourselves and forgetting others.

When we are self-dependent, responsible, free of inner or outer constraints and appropriately active, then we can experience our own true self. We no longer feel the need to dominate or control someone else, we don't manipulate, we won't have to be self-centred and disregard others. We know who we are. We are able not only to hear but also to listen, we allow the other person their own humanness and we won't try to change them into the way we think they should be. We will try to change ourselves, which after all is all we can change and that is no easy task.

Different people go through life in different ways. Some people do what they want to do, some people do what they need to do, some people do what they think others want them to do. It is possible to do what you choose to do out of a feeling for what is right.

12. Humanness

We were born to be human, with unique capacities that are solely man's. Hands to create with, a brain to think with, a heart to love with. Our hands can cause destruction or create beauty, our brain can think how to destroy the world or how to understand it and care for it, our heart can be jealous and destructive or warm and loving. The choice is ours. Because we have been given the ability to choose, we are able to be free, free to love or free to destroy.

The child is born with a trust in those who care for him, he brings with him a feeling of wonder and awe and reverence. How can we keep alive these human qualities? These are qualities that we were all born with. Have we kept them alive in ourselves? We are tempted by the machines to be inactive, we are surrounded by a synthetic world that does not respond to us, money has assumed such importance that we are working ourselves to death to have enough of it. Mothers are off working, homes stand empty all day long, while the people who wanted the home are off trying to earn enough money to pay for it. The very things that we are willing to work for, we are unable to enjoy. If both parents are working to have a home, then they cannot be there to care for it and make it humanly beautiful. Children are cared for in nurseries by a rotating staff that can hardly be expected to create a familiar path for an individual child. What are our priorities?

Have we progressed to be a more civilized nation, a world power? Do we have the wisdom to tell other countries how to order their lives? We daily witness man's inhumanity to man, the destruction of our environment and consequently our health. Are we on a predetermined collision course or can we choose another path? Is the life that we are leading what we really choose to live, or are we caught up in a current that is carrying us along despite our own values?

We do have the capacity to choose, to maintain a balance between the two extremes that are destructive to man and to the world, to shape it in the way that allows us to be human and allows our children to live with dignity and learn of freedom and responsibility. We can choose to live in a world that will allow children to unfold the gifts that they have brought, to understand the world and care for it, not merely use it. We can know truth and reality and bring love and wisdom.

All this is possible, but it won't happen automatically, not by wishful thinking or by trusting that someone else will turn the world around. It is up to parents, to each of us to be the models for our children; to allow children to manifest their God-given gifts. Will we turn our children into clever robots and robot operators or will we allow them to be human, to feel, understand, create and to love?

Our values, our choices, how we spend our time with our children, is what will make the difference. That is the basis of the environment that we create.

In general we don't need our children in the way they were needed in pioneer times. What we do need is the qualities of children to live in the world. Each child can manifest these if we value childhood enough to allow children to be children. Their trust, and awe, their wonder and reverence, their love and acceptance remind us what it means to be human. We shall stop long enough to really look and really listen to what children have to tell us and not be in a hurry to turn their human qualities into cleverness. For what purpose? To impress our friends? What is the real value to the child of five, four or three learning to read? Yes, we can do it, in some cases, but why?

While we are shaping him into a clever man-made premature adult, what are we taking away from him and the world? What are we missing? What will happen to his capacities for creativity that are nurtured by imagination and inner discovery? There is great wisdom in the fairy tales that can be read to the child, but if we are spending the time teaching him to read, he will miss the fairy tales. By the time he is able to read well enough to read the fairy tales, his inner need for them will have passed. Through children's games, and songs and rhymes, spatial concepts are learned in a natural imaginative, subconscious way. 'London bridge is *falling down*', '*round* and *round* the mulberry bush', '*over* the candle stick', incorporates dimensions in the child's experience and vocabulary without becoming isolated concepts. His world stays whole.

From children we can learn to play again, to live in and enjoy the moment, neither worrying about the past nor fearing the future. We can be reminded of the importance of doing what we are doing, while we are doing it. We cannot find a better example of concentration than a child who is totally absorbed in what he is doing, nor a better example of courage than a child learning to walk. Look for these qualities in your children and be reminded that those are your qualities too. If somehow they have become lost or tarnished, join your child in his world and let them grow in you again.

In turn provide for your child the path he needs to find his way into the world, allow him to live in a consistent, protected, rhythmic environment, with form, not chaos, with family rituals, with natural substances, in contact with nature. Allow him to be an apprentice to learn how to care for himself and others, and care for the world.

What is in his environment, what is outer when he is a child will become inner experiences and will help form his personality and develop his character. The personality and character that will become his instrument to meet the world as an adult. Be selective about his environment, remembering that everything matters. Have faith in the child and know how forgiving he will be of our errors as long as our intention is to care for him in the way that is right for him. Remember the trust and warmth that were gifts from birth, and care for those qualities. What we do, and how we do it, are important.

When the child lives with parents who care for the things that they use in the world, the child will have a built-in sense of human values. He will not value the object more than the person. He will learn to appreciate the people who have made the things he uses. He will see the object in relation to himself and the other people that made it. Then feelings of isolation and separateness will fade away. Admiration for cleverness and arrogance will be replaced by a true understanding of man, of his humanness and the humanness in all mankind.

Cold-hearted contempt, criticism, and prejudice will be replaced by warm-hearted understanding, caring, real listening, evaluating, and compassion. As the warm sun melts the cold ice, rounds it and softens it; so can human warmth melt away the separateness and isolation, greed and selfishness that exist in the world.

Whatever we give to a machine to do, we take away from a person. Every time. Let us be certain that when we give a machine a man's task, we really want to replace that man's activity with a machine's activity.

We are eliminating human labour from farms, by developing machines to replace the men. Then the agribusiness develops crops to please the machines, not the people that are eating the food. Strawberries that are solid and tasteless, tomatoes that are solid and tasteless, all for what purpose? Not because no one wants to work on farms. We have unemployed farm workers who know that caring for the land and crops is one of man's most important tasks. But we have taken their jobs away and given them to machines and we have ended up with inferior tasting fruits and vegetables, plus growing unemployment.

Do we really know what we are doing? What price are we willing to pay for showing how clever we can be? Is that the choice that we want to make?

It is easy to fall into thinking in terms of progress without realizing the consequences to the people in the world. While thinking about freedom and equality, we may forget about brotherhood. We need to make human decisions considering all mankind, not just our own personal interests. Decisions need to include what is right for man, not only what is right for the economics of the world. When we give money a reality that does not belong to it and then make that non-reality into a dictator, we have gone a long way down the path of world destruction and self-destruction. Man is free to choose if he wants to care for the world and the people in it or if he wants to destroy it. Know what choice you are making for yourself and for others. Know what world you are creating for your children.

What is good and what is bad is not inherent in the things themselves, but it is in man's use of things. We can use fire to warm a home, cook a meal, soften metals so that they can be formed into useful items, or we can use fire to destroy: to burn down buildings, to defoliate, destroy forests. The evil is in man's choice and action, not in the element of fire. The choices are ours and the choices that we make determine what kind of world we provide for our children. We can use any of the elements — fire, water, or air — constructively or destructively. We need balance in all things, too much or too little will be harmful.

Before we use our cleverness to straighten rivers,

and change the flow of water, we had better first have a deep understanding of nature and understand the consequences of our action. Why are natural water flows, streams, rivers, creeks, always curved? What happens when water moves in curves and spirals? Rivers that have been straightened slowly become polluted, fish die, birds leave. When allowed to return to their natural course, they become alive again. Fish and birds live there again. Nature has many things to tell us if we learn to listen, to observe and to understand rather than trying to control nature with clever ideas.

When a child can find out for himself that blue paint and yellow paint turn to green paint where they meet, he has the experience of inner discovery. How different that is from memorizing the information that blue and yellow make green. When a child can observe, experience and find out the magic of the world through inner discovery, he develops the capacity to experience reality. The child who has had the experience of discovering green will perhaps one day look at the yellow sun, the blue sky and blue river, and wonder about the green grass and green trees. Experiences of wonder are real nourishment for children. Being in the presence of people he can respect and look up to with awe are also necessary food for children. Children need wonder. When we give quick clever explanations about the world we deprive the child of an important experience. The feeling of wonder is a gift that needs to be protected. It may be easy to give glib answers of explanation, but that does not lead to understanding. Interest in the world is enhanced by the feeling of wonder. Experiencing wonder, reverence and respect allow the human qualities in the child to become alive. Later this can develop into a sense of responsibility for the world.

Every time we put a safety device on something we take away part of man's responsibility and a chance to use his consciousness. We think we can make things so safe that it does not matter what we do. We build in automatic safeguards and take away from human responsibility.

What kind of twisted thinking has led to the idea that infants (even those too young to crawl) should not have clothing made out of natural cotton material? Is it thinking, or merchandizing, advertising, and lobbying by the petrochemical companies? Certainly we don't want unnecessary dangers for our children, but what are the limits to safety? What about the pollutants from synthetics? What about all their other clothes? Certainly we don't intend to make the world so 'safe' that a mother does not have to watch her child, care for him, know where he is. The child needs to learn about the law of nature that fire burns if it is not used with caution.

When we can do things unconsciously because they are so safe that they don't require our attention, we create boredom. Ask the man in the automated assembly line.

When your thinking and your actions are both focussed on the same thing, you do not become bored. When you can do anything without consciousness you are depriving yourself of part of your humanness and you can become bored. Will we continue to accept all the mechanical refinements created to make a profit for the companies that come up with them? Will we let the cleverness continue to creep into our homes and take away our activity and our consciousness? Many high-quality items are produced that do not have gimmicks incorporated in them, that allow us to be human as they help us with our daily tasks. We just need to be awake to what we are buying and select with awareness; to know that the environment we are creating for our family is in tune with the beat of the drum that we hear.

Let us be consistent in what we think is important and what we say we want, and what we are actually doing. We don't feel comfortable and neither do our children when we are saying one thing and doing another. When our thinking, our feeling and our actions are in harmony, chances are we will feel whole and will be providing our child with the environment that will nourish physical and mental health.

As much as possible keep the child's life whole. Let healthy living be part of our daily lives. Have you noticed the family that drives to the park to get exercise? What ever happened to walking, and skating, running, and having a tree to climb? The same with our need for crafts. We buy our clothes, then look for some needlework project to do. Why not make your own and your children's clothes and embroider them?

We frequently know what is missing in our lives and then set up an artificial solution. We take a job that allows for no exercise and then we join a health club. We can get back to choosing a life-style for ourselves that allows us to do all the things in our daily tasks that we know we need for good health. Jobs that let us be creative and active in our primary living experience, not after work and in spare time. We know it is not easy and it will take some turning around to bring things back to reason. We also know many young parents who have done this very thing. They saw the inevitable consequences of continuing the artificial, clever life-style and they did not want it for themselves or their children.

There are a lot of us who know what matters and what is real. If each of us will live it, we can make it real for the world. Children will have the chance to be children, to use their bodies and their imagination, to discover, and when they are grown, they will be responsible, caring adults. Man will have a hand in the future of the world, he will care for nature, learn to understand it and make the world beautiful.

Karl König

Brothers and Sisters

From birth we are under a hidden law that influences our relationship with the world, but it is so basic that we may not even notice it. It is simply our order of birth in the family. The fact of being a first, second or third child determines, according to the author, our encounter with 'people, weather, demands, opportunities and destiny'.

Using examples from life and literature Karl König leads us into secrets about life that will linger on in our minds. We gain insight from him into our most personal relationships and yet at the same time feel our attitude to mankind refreshed and renewed. He also provides a most valuable handbook for any parents who have to cope with the more immediate problems of the family constellation.

Floris Books

Heidi Britz-Crecelius

Children at Play
Preparation for Life

Heidi Britz-Crecelius believes that play is more vital
for the child's future than many parents realize. Her
plea is that children's fantasies should be allowed free
scope, for they are learning through play and the
spontaneous creations of their own magical world.
The more they can be absorbed in their play, from
the earliest joy in little rhythmic movements to the
extended imaginative games of childhood, the more
fully and effectively they later take their place in the
world of adults.

Her book offers many practical suggestions especially for the urban family. Dozens of real children
play through the pages of this book making it a delight
to read and its conclusions convincing. It is a refresh-
ing and a timely warning for a technological age.

Floris Books